AMBULATORY BLOOD PRESSURE RECORDING

AMBULATORY BLOOD PRESSURE RECORDING

Editors

Hans R. Brunner, M.D.
Bernard Waeber, M.D.
Hypertension Division
University Hospital
Lausanne, Switzerland

Raven Press New York

Raven Press, Ltd., 1185 Avenue of the Americas, New York, New York 10036

Made in the United States of America

Library of Congress Cataloging-in-Publication Data

Ambulatory blood pressure recording / edited by Hans Brunner and Bernard Waeber.
p. cm.
Includes bibliographical references and index.
ISBN 0-88167-889-9
1. Ambulatory blood pressure monitoring. I. Brunner, Hans R., 1937–
[DNLM: 1. Blood Pressure Determination—methods. 2. Monitoring, Physiologic. WG 106 A49685]
RC683.5.A43A44
612.1′4—dc20
DNLM/DLC
for Library of Congess 91-43057
CIP

The material contained in this volume was submitted as previously unpublished material, except in the instances in which credit has been given to the source from which some of the illustrative material was derived.

Great care has been taken to maintain the accuracy of the information contained in the volume. However, neither Raven Press nor the editors can be held responsible for errors or for any consequences arising from the use of the information contained herein.

9 8 7 6 5 4 3 2 1

Contents

Contributing Authors

Hans R. Brunner, M.D. *Hypertension Division, University Hospital, 1011 Lausanne, Switzerland*

Edoardo Camenzind, M.D. *Hypertension Division, University Hospital, 1011 Lausanne, Switzerland*

Deanna G. Cheung, M.D. *Department of Medicine, University of California at Irvine, and Hypertension Center, Veterans Administration Medical Center, 5901 East Seventh Avenue, Long Beach, California 90822*

Andrew J. S. Coats, M.D. *Department of Cardiac Medicine, National Heart and Lung Institute, London, SW3 6LY, England*

John Cox, M.D. *Blood Pressure Unit, Beaumont Hospital, Dublin, Ireland*

William F. Graettinger, M.D. *Department of Medicine, University of California at Irvine, and Veterans Administration Medical Center, 5901 East Seventh Avenue, Long Beach, California 90822*

G. Mancia, M.D. *Centro di Fisiologia Clinica e Ipertensione, Ospedale Maggiore, Universitá di Milano, Via F. Sforza 35, Milan 20122, Italy*

E. Mutti, M.D. *Centro di Fisiologia Clinica e Ipertensione, Ospedale Maggiore, Universitá di Milano, Via F. Sforza 35, Milan 20122, Italy*

Joel M. Neutel, M.D. *Department of Medicine, University of California at Irvine, and Hypertension Center, Veterans Administration Medical Center, 5901 East Seventh Avenue, Long Beach, California 90822*

Jürg Nussberger, M.D. *Hypertension Division, University Hospital, 1011 Lausanne, Switzerland*

Eoin O'Brien, M.D. *Blood Pressure Unit, Beaumont Hospital, Dublin, Ireland*

S. Omboni, M.D. *Centro di Fisiologia Clinica e Ipertensione, Ospedale Maggiore, Universitá di Milano, Via F. Sforza 35, Milan 20122, Italy*

G. Parati, M.D. *Centro di Fisologia Clinica e Ipertensione, Ospedale Maggiore, Universitá di Milano, Via F. Sforza 35, Milan 20122, Italy*

Dorothee Perloff, M.D. *Department of Medicine, Division of Cardiology, Moffitt Hospital, University of California at San Francisco, San Francisco, California 94143*

Thomas G. Pickering, M.D., D.Phil. *Cardiovascular Center, The New York Hospital-Cornell University Medical Center, 525 East 68th Street, Starr-4, New York, New York 10021*

Edward Bernard Raftery, M.D., B.Sc., F.A.C.C., F.R.C.P. *MRC Division of Cardiovascular Diseases, Northwick Park Hospital and Clinical Research Center, Watford Road, Harrow, Middlesex HA1 3UJ, England*

Peter Sleight, M.D. *Department of Cardiovascular Medicine, John Radcliffe Hospital, Oxford OX3 9DU, England*

David H. G. Smith, M.D. *Department of Medicine, University of California at Irvine, and Hypertension Center, Veterans Administration Medical Center, 5901 East Seventh Avenue, Long Beach, California 90822*

Maurice Sokolow, M.D. *Department of Medicine, Cardiovascular Research Institute, University of California at San Francisco, San Francisco, California 94143*

Bernard Waeber, M.D. *Hypertension Division, University Hospital, 1011 Lausanne, Switzerland*

Michael A. Weber, M.D. *Department of Internal Medicine, University of California at Irvine, and Hypertension Center, Veterans Administration Medical Center, 5901 East Seventh Avenue, Long Beach, California 90822*

Preface

Diagnosis and treatment of hypertension is traditionally based on blood pressure readings taken by a doctor. There are many good reasons to rely on such readings. They are a valuable indicator of the cardiovascular risk and longterm reduction of these blood pressure readings has been shown to markedly diminish the occurrence of cardiovascular complications. Why then is there a need to reappraise this well-established way of determining blood pressure since most doctors see nothing wrong with the conventional approach. In this respect, they are partly right. It is fair to say that they should continue to use the office blood pressure measurement as a routine procedure. However, keep in mind that blood pressure is a highly variable parameter. For example, blood pressure often rises considerably when the patient faces the doctor; and it responds to various physical and mental activities with great changes. It is now understood that one punctual determination carried out in an unusual environment may not closely reflect one's usual blood pressure.

The pronounced variablity of blood pressure first became apparent when pressure was monitored intra-arterially. A rapidly growing interest has emerged for the non-invasive recording of ambulatory blood pressure as illustrated in the figure below. The number of

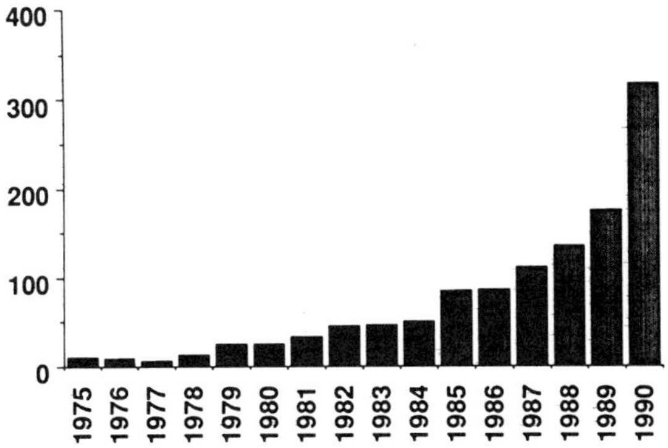

Number of publications on ambulatory blood pressure measurement.

publications dealing with this topic showed a constant progression from 1975 to 1990. Does it mean that the clinical usefulness of this new method of measuring blood pressure is now firmly established? One has to admit that the answer is still no. There is nevertheless circumstantial evidence that suggests non-invasive ambulatory blood pressure monitoring represents a valuable tool for doctors.

This book reviews the problems linked to the different methods of measuring blood pressure. It appears that office and ambulatory recorded blood pressures should be regarded as complementary. This important issue has been critically addressed by all experts having contributed to this book. We believe that this book will be very interesting to any physician involved with blood pressure measurement.

Bernard Waeber, M.D.
Hans R. Brunner, M.D.

Acknowledgment

We would like to express our thanks to all of our friends who helped to summarize the present knowledge on ambulatory blood pressure monitoring.

AMBULATORY BLOOD PRESSURE RECORDING

Ambulatory Blood Pressure Recording,
edited by H. Brunner and B. Waeber.
Raven Press, Ltd., New York © 1992.

1

Problems with Therapeutic Conclusions Based on Intervention Trials

*Andrew J. S. Coats and †Peter Sleight

**Department of Cardiac Medicine, National Heart and Lung Institute, London, SW3 6LY, England and †Department of Cardiovascular Medicine, John Radcliffe Hospital, Oxford, OX3 9DU, England*

A clear positive relationship exists between the level of blood pressure taken on a single occasion and the eventual risk of cardiovascular mortality and morbidity (13,14,21,28,32). Large antihypertensive intervention trials have documented significant reductions in both cardiovascular morbidity and mortality (1,19,20,39,40). Other trials have not shown significant benefits (17,26,27,37,38). The protection against fatal cerebrovascular events is close to that expected given the epidemiologically observed risk and the achieved blood pressure reduction (7). The major killer in hypertension remains, however, coronary-related deaths, and for these the achieved protection appears to be possibly less than that predicted (7) (Fig. 1).

Several questions arise, therefore, in translating these studies into clinical practice: (a) Why is the reduction in coronary related mortality less than expected? (b) At what level in mild blood pressure elevation is antihypertensive treatment warranted? (c) Can we accurately compare the reduction in mortality produced by different antihypertensive regimens?

(a) Many factors that could account for the apparently disappointing reduction in coronary-related mortality have been described. These include a possible adverse effect of treatment on another risk factor for coronary-related death (27), insufficient duration of blood

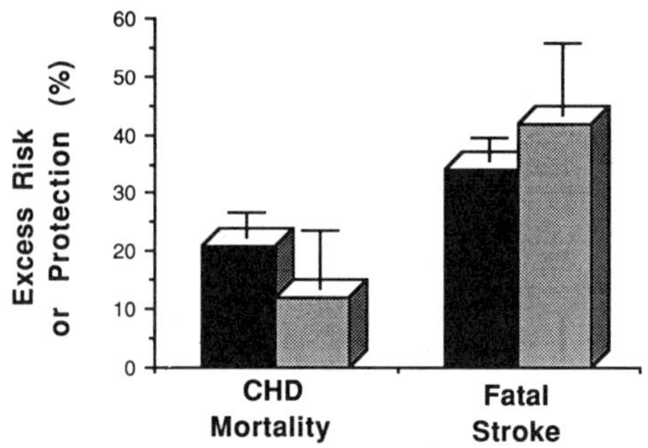

FIG. 1. Bar graph showing the excess risk (*black*) associated with prolonged differences in diastolic blood pressure (DBP) of 5 mm Hg, and the protection from risk (*shaded*) associated with short-term reductions in usual DBP of 5 mmHg achieved by antihypertensive therapy. Data from ref. 7. Bars represent 95% confidence intervals.

pressure reduction (7), or an adverse effect on coronary-related death from too great a reduction in pressure in some subjects (the so-called J-curve) (2,10).

(b) The trials of mortality with treatment in mild hypertension have shown either no or only very small but significant reductions in mortality (17,19,26,27,33,37,40) and there is no consensus on what level of pressure to treat. Part of this uncertainty may relate to the problems of classifying blood pressure on the basis of a few clinic estimates of pressure at trial entry only.

(c) The large intervention trials were based on treatments including predominantly diuretic or antiadrenergic agents and many newer agents are now advocated for the treatment of hypertension. The cost and ethics of studying even a representative agent from each group in the large prolonged trials necessary to prove beneficial effects on mortality reduction would be significant. There will always remain, however, doubts about whether blood pressure reduction is always associated with mortality reduction with newer agents, so that efforts to prove benefit will be necessary. Even the comparison in quantitative blood pressure reduction between different agents is difficult and most published trials are not powerful enough to detect even quite large differences between agents (16). Ambulatory monitoring may help in this regard by increasing the accuracy of estimates of risk and blood pressure reduction (6,8).

The ability to better classify subjects and to more accurately follow blood pressure over time may make mortality trials with newer agents feasible with fewer patients.

The following discussion will concentrate on the role of ambulatory pressure monitoring in addressing the problems described above, and in deriving improved therapeutic guidelines.

CLINIC OR AMBULATORY BLOOD PRESSURE DETERMINATION AS THE BASIS FOR TRIALS

Most of the major epidemiological studies of blood pressure, and the major interventional blood pressure lowering trials have based their conclusions on only one, two, or three measurements of blood pressure in a clinical setting at trial entry only. The inaccuracies inherent in estimates of blood pressure based on a few clinic readings are well known and include an underestimation of risk by a "regression dilution" bias (3,12,23), and imprecision in estimating hypotensive effects because of the high variability of these measurements (5). Systematic overestimation of pressure by clinic measurements occur in about 20 to 30% of subjects (15,18,22,24,31) ("white-coat" hypertension) who may, consequently, be misdiagnosed as hypertensive and receive inappropriate pressure reduction (22,41), which could dilute or even reverse the effect of treatment on risk.

Ambulatory pressure monitoring is both more reproducible (5,6) and more closely related to mortality and morbidity (29,30) than clinic blood pressure. Ambulatory monitoring also helps identify and exclude from trials "white-coat" hypertensives who only have elevated blood pressures in the clinic or office setting (31,41).

THE BLOOD PRESSURE:RISK RELATIONSHIP

The major epidemiological surveys have established the adverse risk associated with elevated clinic blood pressure (13,14,21, 28,32).

The J-Curve

The relation between risk and pressure level is not as clear-cut at the lower end of the blood pressure distribution, and it has been suggested that there is a J- or U-shaped curve with increasing risk as blood pressure (usually measured as diastolic) falls below a certain low value (2,10,11); this was originally suggested by Stewart (36) from a long-term audit of his own practice.

The number of deaths or cardiovascular events in this blood pressure range is, however, small, and it is much more difficult to prove statistically the shape of the curve in this range (7). Other factors that may contribute to a J shape include: other diseases associated with increased mortality producing weight loss and blood pressure reduction in the months leading up to death; established arterial disease with increased large arterial stiffness producing a selective reduction in diastolic blood pressure (35); and the use of treatments for established coronary artery disease that secondarily lower blood pressure.

Combining the results of the major population surveys MacMahon et al. (23) have recently presented convincing statistical evidence on over 400,000 subjects that there was a continuous positive relation between diastolic blood pressure (DBP) and risk of death with no evidence for a J-shaped tail at the lower end of the pressure distribution.

Most of the suggestive evidence for a J-curve relates to trials with a high incidence of subjects with coronary artery disease. It is not clear whether overzealous pharmacological lowering of DBP may have an adverse effect on coronary blood flow and hence indirectly on mortality (11), or whether subjects with stiff arteries (and low DBP because of this) and coronary artery disease are already subject to a poorer prognosis because of these factors, rather than as a result of a low DBP (35). In the large Multiple Risk Factor Intervention Trial (MRFIT) (34), in which 360,000 people were screened, it can be seen that for a given low systolic pressure both systolic and diastolic pressures are positively related to future risk, whereas with a higher systolic pressure (> 160 mm Hg) the highest risk occurs at the lowest diastolic pressures suggesting that the relation might be with stiff arteries rather than diastolic BP per se (Fig. 2) (35).

No trial or analysis, however, has been large enough to determine beyond doubt if pressure can be lowered too far, so that the J-curve remains hypothetical, and cannot be used as a basis for guiding treatment of the hypertensive population at large.

Regression Dilution

It has recently been reemphasized that the steepness of the pressure:risk relationship is underestimated quite significantly if risk is related to initial blood pressure alone (23). Because of the tendency of subpopulation means to regress toward the total population mean (3,12), there is a closer and steeper relationship between risk and

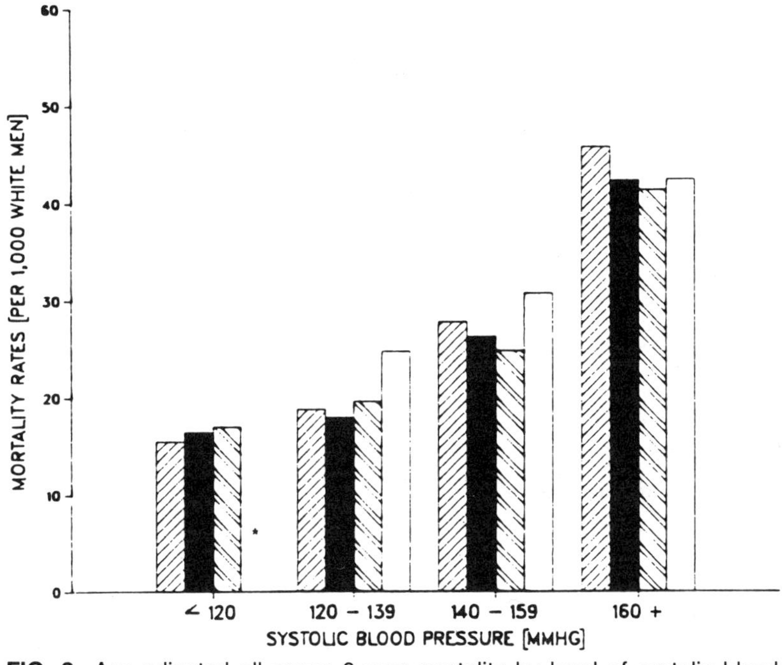

FIG. 2. Age-adjusted all-cause 6-year mortality by level of systolic blood pressure (SBP) and DBP for white Multiple Risk Factor Intervention Trial (MRFIT) screenees (age 35 to 57 at initial screening). ▨, DBP < 80 mmHG; ■, DBP 80–89 mmHG; ▧ DBP 90–99 mmHG; □ DBP 100+ mmHG. (Reproduced from ref. 34 with permission.)

the average of in-study blood pressure than for initial or entry blood pressure; this has been coined the "regression dilution" bias (23) (Fig. 3). From analyzing in-study pressures from the Framingham study MacMahon et al. (23) estimated a 60% steeper slope than for entry pressures; when relative risk is expressed on a doubling scale the relationship with pressure is close to linear.

Another way of obtaining the relationship between "true" or usual

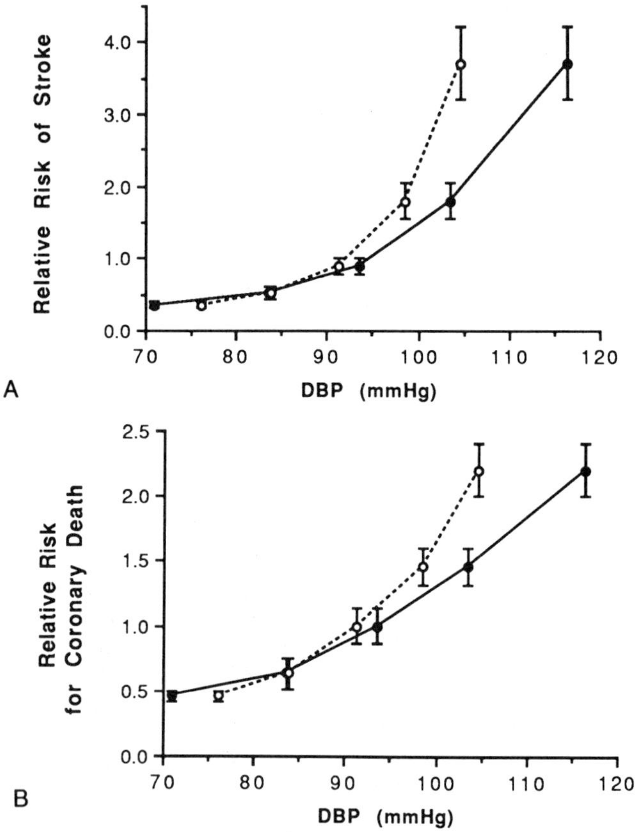

FIG. 3. A: Relative risk of stroke against initial and usual diastolic blood pressures. Redrawn from the data of the Framingham study as presented in ref. 23. **B:** Relative risks of coronary-related deaths against initial and usual DBP. (Redrawn from ref. 23.) *Filled circles, solid line* represents initial DBP and *open circles, dotted line* represents usual DBP. Bars represent 95% confidence intervals for relative risks.

pressure and risk is by mathematical correction of the entry pressure:risk slope if the intermeasurement correlation is known (3,12). Such analysis using our own data (see next section) agrees that the steepness of the true slope would be over 60% greater than observed for a single entry estimate of pressure. The interpretation of conventional data has, therefore, quite markedly underestimated the true importance of minor elevations of blood pressure maintained over a long period.

Ambulatory Monitoring and Regression Dilution

It is not always feasible or desirable to measure pressures over many years before determining the usual level of pressure, and ambulatory monitoring may give a much more accurate estimate of usual BP after one record than would a single or duplicate estimate of pressure in the clinic. Our data on reproducibility and interestimate correlations of clinic and ambulatory pressures can be used to calculate the degree of regression dilution for the two methods, and regression to the mean can be investigated directly from similar data. Analyzed either way ambulatory recordings can be shown to be far less subject to regression to the mean than clinic BP estimates, and might, therefore, give a much more precise pressure:risk slope if a population survey using this method of recording were to be conducted. The presence of large but clinically unpredictable (15) alerting responses in some subjects makes it even more important for this information to be obtained (25,31).

In our clinic we have looked at the 1-month reproducibility of clinic and ambulatory pressure estimates in a large number of untreated subjects with a wide range of blood pressures (6) (Fig. 4). We have also shown how reduced variability and increased intermonth correlation depends on the number of readings per day (8) (Table 1). Subdividing our subjects into the same pressure quintiles as the Framingham data we can compare long-term regression to the mean with what we found over 1 month for clinic and ambulatory readings (Table 2). It is clear that ambulatory recordings are much less subject to regression dilution, and this should allow much more accurate risk estimation for a given ambulatory pressure. Clearly what is

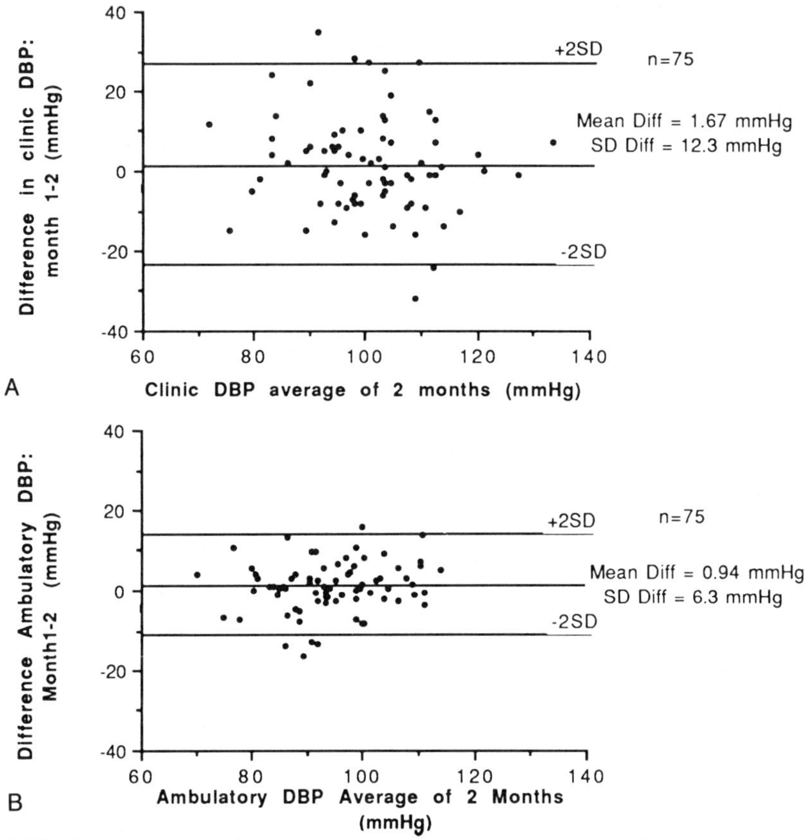

FIG. 4. Bland-Altman plots showing the repeatability of clinic **(A)** and ambulatory **(B)** DBP after 1 month in 75 untreated hypertensive subjects. (Reproduced from ref. 9 with permission.)

needed is a population survey of ambulatory pressures (4,42) to plot this relationship directly, as it is well known that ambulatory pressure is usually (but not predictably) significantly lower than clinic pressure for individual subjects.

INTERPRETATION OF INTERVENTION TRIALS

Intervention trials are divided into two main types: the large long-term trial with mortality or morbidity reduction as a desired end-

TABLE 1. *Repeatability of diastolic blood pressure after 1 month*

	SDD[a] (mm Hg)	Intermonth correlation (r value)
Clinic reading	12.6	.59
1 ambulatory reading	13.8	.51
2 ambulatory readings	10.4	.66
4 ambulatory readings	8.8	.73
8 ambulatory readings	8.3	.75
>20 ambulatory readings	6.5	.83

[a]Standard deviations of difference (SDD) and month 1 to month 2 correlations of diastolic blood pressure based on clinic reading or increasing numbers of readings from a daytime period of ambulatory monitoring in 100 subjects.

TABLE 2. *Regression to the mean for diastolic blood pressure: comparing the Framingham remeasurements after 4 years, with remeasurement of clinic and ambulatory DBP after 1 month in 100 subjects*

	Mean DBP change (regression to the mean)[a]		
	Framingham	Clinic	Ambulatory
DBP ≤79 mmHg	+5.4	–[b]	–
DBP 80–89 mmHg	+0.3	+2.2	+2.1
DBP 90–99 mmHg	−2.2	+1.3	−0.3
DBP 100–109 mmHg	−4.9	−1.8	−2.1
DBP ≥ 110 mmHg	−11.7	−13.5	−1.8

[a]Extents of regressions to the mean for estimates of diastolic blood pressure for subjects in arbitrary blood pressure groups on the first reading. The table shows the size of the regression for extremes of pressure and shows that repeat clinic measurements after 1 month reflect only a part of the 4-year regression effect, and that ambulatory recording is considerably less subject to the regression to the mean phenomenon.

[b]Insufficient numbers.

point, and the smaller shorter trial where pressure reduction itself is the endpoint.

The Large Mortality Trials

Attempts at meta-analysis of the controlled long-term intervention trials have shown that for cerebrovascular events the reductions in mortality and morbidity are both statistically highly significant, and clinically important (7). Collins et al. (7) also have recently demonstrated that the achieved reductions in cerebrovascular events are of the magnitude to be expected if most of the adverse risk associated with increased pressure could be abolished by relatively short-term (a few years) reductions in blood pressure by therapy.

The reduction in coronary-related mortality in these trials, however, is about half that expected if all the excess risk of prolonged BP elevation could be abolished by relatively short-term antihypertensive treatment. As Collins et al. (7) point out, however, this may be due to a number of possible factors, one of which is the play of statistical chance. Other explanations have been referred to earlier.

Major trials in mild hypertension show a high proportion of subjects with initially raised blood pressure becoming normotensive with no treatment (1,18,26,33). In the Australian trial in mild hypertension this amounted to 13% of those found to be hypertensive at the screening visits never reaching these levels of blood pressure again throughout the duration of the trial, and for the placebo group 25% of subjects having a mean in-trial diastolic blood pressure below 90 mmHg (33). These effects may be in part due to a combination of regression to the mean and a waning of the clinic alerting response with time. Thus, clinic estimates of blood pressure, which are more subject to such errors, may significantly underestimate the mortality reduction associated with a given mean pressure reduction in the whole trial population. The dual errors of unregressed pressure estimation at entry (they were not really as hypertensive as initially thought) and the inclusion of some "white-coat" hypertensives (they were not really hypertensive at all), make it highly likely that we have missed the full impact on mortality of the treatment of mild elevations of *usual* blood pressure. There is clearly a strong case for attempting trials of mild hypertension using ambulatory monitoring to evaluate entry criteria and treatment effects.

The Small Antihypertensive Trial

As befits the importance of hypertension and its treatment there is a very large literature of relatively small short-term trials of the antihypertensive effects of new drugs, either against placebo or against an established treatment. An unfortunately high proportion of these trials are too small to accurately determine the true average pressure reduction (16), and where active treatments are compared it is very common to be unable to differentiate the agents' abilities to reduce blood pressure. The use of ambulatory pressure monitoring has been shown to dramatically reduce the necessary size of such trials (5,9) or conversely increase the statistical power and decrease the confidence intervals for the hypotensive effect in trials of a given size (6,8). This is illustrated in Fig. 5. It is questionable if

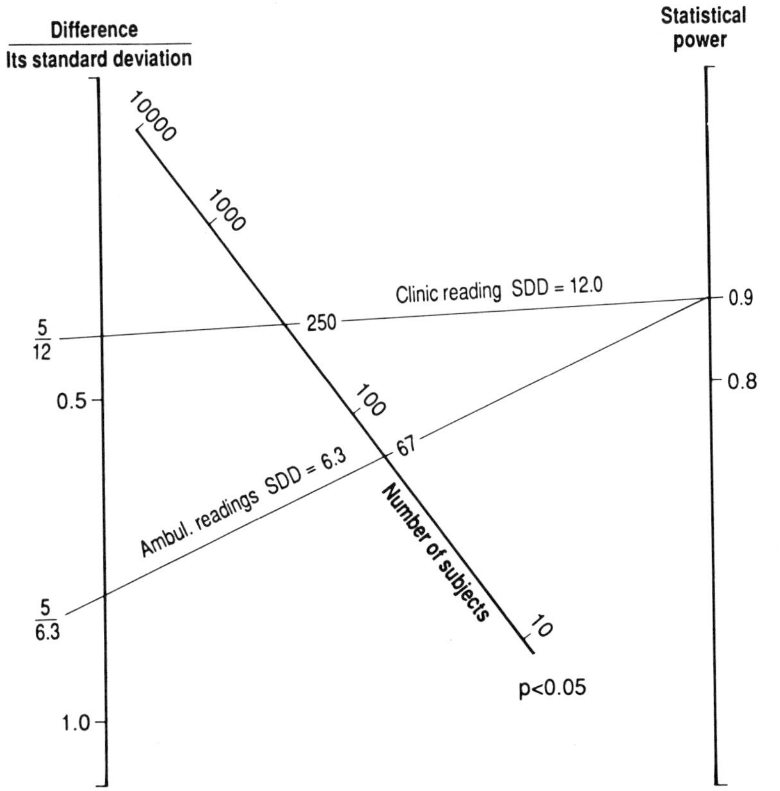

FIG. 5. A nomogram showing how the variability of repeated measurements has a profound effect on the numbers of subjects needed in a parallel group trial. Difference (D), the hypotensive difference in pressure the trial is designed to test for; SDD, the standard deviation of differences of repeat pressure measurements without intervention. Ambulatory monitoring reduces SDD dramatically, thereby increasing the D/SDD ratio and reducing subject number for the same statistical power. (Reproduced from ref. 9 with permission.)

the continued use of large numbers of subjects in antihypertensive trials in which pressure estimation is by clinic measurement alone is justifiable given the very large variability, and misdiagnosis rate of this method (8).

CONCLUSIONS

Large epidemiological trials have told us a lot about the risks of prolonged blood pressure elevation, but we have probably still underestimated the risk because of a regression dilution bias. For coronary-related deaths the full potential benefit of therapeutic blood pressure reduction has not been achieved, but the precise reason for this is uncertain. Many intervention trials, both large and small, have been marred by depending solely on clinic blood pressure estimates.

The increasing availability and acceptance of ambulatory monitoring may finally allow a more accurate description of the risk of usual blood pressure levels, and would certainly increase the precision of intervention trials. Prospective epidemiological and intervention trials with ambulatory monitoring thus hold the potential to determine if and why coronary-related death is not being adequately avoided by hypotensive treatment, and may allow us to draw up more accurate therapeutic guidelines for different levels of usual blood pressure. Such trials would also be much better able to detect differences between alternative drug regimes, which have hitherto been obscured by trials both too small and too imprecise.

REFERENCES

1. Amery A, Birkenhäger W, Brixko P, Bulpitt C, Clement D, Deruyttere M, De Schaepdryver A, Dollery C, Fagard R, Forette F, Forte J, Hamdy R, Henry JF, Joossens JV, Leonetti G, Lund-Johansen P, O'Malley K, Petrie J, Strasser T, Tuomilehto J, Williams B. Mortality and morbidity results from the European Working Party on High Blood Pressure in the Elderly trial. *Lancet* 1985;1:1349–1354.
2. Anderson TW. Re-examination of some of the Framingham blood-pressure data. *Lancet* 1978;2:1139–1141.
3. Berkson J. Are there two regressions? *J Am Stat Assoc* 1950;45:164–180.

4. Brunner HR. Concluding remarks. *J Hypertens* 1989;7(suppl 3):S109.
5. Coats AJS, Conway J, Somers VK, Isea JE, Sleight P. Ambulatory pressure monitoring in the assessment of antihypertensive therapy. *Cardiovasc Drug Therapy* 1989;3:303–311.
6. Coats AJS, Radaelli A, Clark S, Conway J, Sleight P. The influence of ambulatory blood pressure monitoring on the design and interpretation of trials in hypertension. *J Hypertens* (in press)
7. Collins R, Peto R, MacMahon S, Hebert P, Fiebach NH, Eberlein KA, Qilizbash N, Taylor JO, Hennekens CH. Effects of short-term reductions in diastolic blood pressure on stroke and coronary heart disease: evidence from an overview of randomised drug trials considered in the context of observational epidemiology. *Lancet* 1990;335:827–838.
8. Conway J, Coats A. Value of ambulatory blood pressure monitoring in clinical pharmacology. *J Hypertens* 1989;7(suppl 3):S29–S32.
9. Conway J, Johnston J, Coats A, Somers V, Sleight P. The use of ambulatory blood pressure monitoring to improve the accuracy and reduce the numbers of subjects in clinical trials of antihypertensive agents. *J Hypertens* 1988;6:111–116.
10. Cruickshank JM. Coronary blood flow and the J curve relation between diastolic blood pressure and myocardial infarction. *Br Med J* 1988;297:1227–1230.
11. Cruickshank JM, Thorp JM, Zacharias FJ. Benefits and potential harm of lowering high blood pressure. *Lancet* 1987;1:581–584.
12. Davis CE. The effect of regression to the mean in epidemiologic and clinical studies. *Am J Epidemiol* 1976;104:493–498.
13. Dawber TR. *The Framingham study. The epidemiology of atherosclerotic disease*. Cambridge: Harvard University Press, 1980.
14. Dyer AR. An analysis of the relationship of systolic blood pressure, serum cholesterol, and smoking to 14-year mortality in the Chicago People's Gas Company study—II. Coronary and cardiovascular-renal mortality in two competing risk models. *J Chron Dis* 1975;28:571–578.
15. Floras JS, Jones JV, Hassan MO, Osikowska B, Sever PS, Sleight P. Cuff and ambulatory blood pressure in subjects with essential hypertension. *Lancet* 1981;1:107–109.
16. Freestone S, Silas JH, Ramsay LE. Sample size for short-term trials of antihypertensive drugs. *Br J Clin Pharmacol* 1982;14:265–268.
17. Helgeland A. Treatment of mild hypertension: a five year controlled drug trial. The Oslo study. *Am J Med* 1980;69:725–732.
18. Hense HW, Keil U. The effect of multiple and repeated blood pressure measurements on the diagnosis of hypertension. Results of the Munich blood pressure study I and the Munich blood pressure programme (Abstract). *J Hypertens* 1985;3:414–415.
19. Hypertension Detection and Follow-up Program Cooperative Group. Five-year findings of the hypertension detection and follow-up program. I. Reduction in mortality of persons with high blood pressure, including mild hypertension. *JAMA* 1979;242:2562–2571.
20. Hypertension Detection and Follow-up Program Cooperative Group. Five-year findings of the hypertension detection and follow-up program. III. Reduction in stroke incidence among persons with high blood pressure. *JAMA* 1982;247:633–638.

21. Kagan A, Harris BR, Winkelstein W Jr, Johnson KG, Kato H, Syme SL, Rhoads GG, Gay ML, Nichaman NZ, Hamilton HB, Tillotson J. Epidemiologic studies of coronary heart disease and stroke in Japanese men living in Japan, Hawaii and California: demographic, physical, dietary and biochemical characteristics. *J Chron Dis* 1974;27:345–364.
22. Krakoff LR, Eison H, Phillips RH, Leiman SJ, Lev S. Effect of ambulatory blood pressure monitoring on the diagnosis and cost of treatment for mild hypertension. *Am Heart J* 1988;116:1152–1154.
23. MacMahon S, Peto R, Cutler R, Collins R, Sorlie P, Neaton J, Abbott R, Godwin J, Dyer A, Stamler J. Effects of prolonged differences in diastolic blood pressure on the risks of stroke and of coronary heart disease. *Lancet* 1990;335:765–774.
24. Mancia G, Parati G, Pomidossi G, Grassi G, Casadei R, Zanchetti A. Alerting reaction and rise in blood pressure during measurement by physician and nurse. *Hypertension* 1987;9:209–215.
25. McCall WC, McCall VR. Diagnostic use of ambulatory blood pressure monitoring in medical practice. *J Fam Pract* 1981;13:25–30.
26. Medical Research Council Working Party. MRC trial of treatment of mild hypertension: principal results. *Br Med J* 1985;291:97–104.
27. Multiple Risk Factor Intervention Trial Research Group. Multiple risk factor intervention trial: risk factor changes and mortality results. *JAMA* 1982;248: 1465–1477.
28. Neaton JD, Kuller LH, Wentworth D, Borhani NO. Total and cardiovascular mortality in relation to cigarette smoking, serum cholesterol concentration, and diastolic blood pressure among black and white males followed up for five years. *Am Heart J* 1984;108:759–769.
29. Perloff D, Sokolow M, Cowan R. The prognostic value of ambulatory blood pressures. *JAMA* 1983;249:2792–2798.
30. Perloff D, Sokolow M, Cowan RM, Juster RP. Prognostic value of ambulatory blood pressure measurements: further analysis. *J Hypertens* 1989;7(suppl 3): S3–S10.
31. Pickering TG, James GD. Some implications of the differences between home, clinic and ambulatory blood pressure in normotensive and hypertensive patients. *J Hypertens* 1989;7(suppl 3):S65–S72.
32. Reid DD, McCartney P, Hamilton PJS, Rose G. Smoking and other risk factors for coronary heart-disease in British civil servants. *Lancet* 1976;2:979–984.
33. Report by the Management Committee. The Australian therapeutic trial in mild hypertension. *Lancet* 1980;1:1261–1267.
34. Rutan GH, Kuller LH, Neaton JD, Wentworth DN, McDonald RH, McFate Smith W. Mortality associated with diastolic hypertension and isolated systolic hypertension among men screened for the Multiple Risk Factor Intervention Trial. *Circulation* 1988;77:504–514.
35. Sleight P. Pressures, hearts and U-shaped curves. *Lancet* 1988;1:235.
36. Stewart IMcDG. Relation of reduction in pressure to first myocardial infarction in patients receiving treatment for severe hypertension. *Lancet* 1979;1: 861–865.
37. The IPPPSH Collaborative Group. Cardiovascular risk and risk factors in a randomized trial of treatment based on the beta-blocker oxprenolol: The Inter-

national Prospective Primary Prevention Study in Hypertension (IPPPSH). *J Hypertens* 1985;3:379–392.
38. US Public Health Service Hospitals Cooperative Study Group. Treatment of mild hypertension: results of a ten-year intervention trial. *Circ Res* 1977;40 (Suppl 1):98–105.
39. Veterans Administration Cooperative Study Group on Antihypertensive Agents. Effects of treatment on morbidity in hypertension. Results in patients with diastolic blood pressures averaging 115 through 129 mm Hg. *JAMA* 1967;202:1028–1034.
40. Veterans Administration Cooperative Study Group on Antihypertensive Agents. Effects of treatment on morbidity in hypertension. II. Results in patients with diastolic blood pressures averaging 90 through 114 mm Hg. *JAMA* 1970;213:1143–1152.
41. Waeber B, Scherrer U, Petrillo A, Bidiville J, Nussberger J, Waeber G, Hofstetter J-R, Brunner HR. Are some hypertensive patients overtreated? A prospective study of ambulatory blood pressure recording. *Lancet* 1987;2: 732–734.
42. Weber MA. Evaluating the diagnosis and prognosis of hypertension by automated blood pressure monitoring: outline of a symposium. *Am Heart J* 1988; 116:1118–1123.

Ambulatory Blood Pressure Recording,
edited by H. Brunner and B. Waeber.
Raven Press, Ltd., New York © 1992.

2

From Invasive to Non-Invasive Ambulatory Blood Pressure Recording

Edward Bernard Raftery

Division of Cardiovascular Diseases, Northwick Park Hospital and Clinical Research Center, Middlesex, HA1 3UJ, England

A well-known radio philosopher and pundit of the 1940s, Professor C.E.M. Joad, used to preface his remarks with the statement: "It all depends upon what you mean by . . ." It is a matter of record that none of the authors of the numerous books and monographs on blood pressure have defined what it is they are trying to measure. Even the incomparable physiologist Carl Wiggers offered no definition: only a description of how he measured "it" (36).

Pressure is defined as force per unit area. Therefore, arterial blood pressure should be defined as the lateral forces exerted on the wall of the artery in question whenever the left ventricle contracts and ejects blood into a system that is already full of blood. This definition is inherent in Wiggers' description of how he measured arterial blood pressure: from the sidearm of a brass T-piece with the bar sewn into the lumen of the artery. Because the left ventricle is a discontinuous pump, the pressure events can be expressed as a mean, or as a phasic complex with a maximum (systolic), dependent mainly upon the rate of ejection into a constant elastic-walled system, and a minimum (diastolic), dependent mainly upon the resistance that the peripheral arterioles present to forward flow.

All of this was appreciated, if not expressed, by the 19th century physiologists who first described the techniques for the measurement of arterial blood pressure in animals and humans. The experimental physiologist could expose arteries and insert tubes fitted with membranes and mirrors that would reflect beams of light onto photographic film. The physical characteristics of these systems, and hence the accuracy of the results, could be fully described, and although the techniques were cumbersome and time-consuming, there can be no questioning the validity of the results obtained and the conclusions reached. But the best the human physiologist could hope for was a technique that could give some approximation of the lateral forces without the need for invasive exposure of the vessel itself.

The driving force was the centuries-old appreciation of the relationship between mortality and the perceived tension of the palpated pulse (32). And what evolved was the Riva-Rocci/Korotkoff technique for the measurement of blood pressure, which became part of the routine physical examination 80 years ago, and has remained substantially unchanged ever since.

THE INDIRECT METHOD

The apparatus consists of a cuff that encloses an inflatable bladder, which can be wrapped around the upper arm. The bladder is inflated by means of a small hand-pump, until the pulse below the cuff disappears. The cuff is then allowed to deflate while the observer listens over the brachial artery below the cuff, and the pressure within the bladder is monitored by a mercury-in-glass manometer. When the pressure in the artery above the cuff starts to exceed the pressure within the bladder, the critical opening pressure of the occluded vessel is exceeded, and partial opening occurs with each pulse. This event is accompanied by the appearance of sound (Korotkoff I), and equates to systolic blood pressure. As deflation continues, each pressure pulse achieves greater opening of the occluded vessel until a point is reached when the vessel remains partially open throughout each cardiac cycle. When this happens, the quality of each Korotkoff sound changes with disappearance of high-frequency components (Korotkoff IV, muffling) and this point equates to diastolic pressure. As deflation continues, there comes a point at which the deflated vessel remains fully open throughout each cycle, with the disappearance of sound (Korotkoff V). There is still considerable controversy about whether Korotkoff IV or V properly represents diastolic pressure (28) but for the sake of convenience, V is usually taken. Thus the technique gives an estimate of systolic and diastolic blood pressure over a minimum of 15 beats and under conditions where the subject is still and in a standardized position while the procedure goes forward.

Other indirect techniques have evolved around this basic method, but in every case the principles are the same and the only differences are in the method used to detect wall motion in the occluded brachial artery. Thus, oscillometry, ultrasound, and infrasound are all variations on the same theme and make the same methodological assumptions as the Riva-Rocci/Korotkoff technique.

THE DIRECT METHOD

It is remarkable how little the indirect method of measuring blood pressure has changed in the last 80 years; this is in stark contrast to the direct method. The earliest principle of a high-frequency membrane with a small displacement has been retained, but the technology has become highly sophisticated. It was realized very early that total exposure of a vessel was not necessary if a fluid-filled cannula with the membrane at the outer end could be introduced into the vessel. The advent of the strain-gauge and the progressive miniaturization of the equipment and recording apparatus has completed the revolution, and devices of all levels of sophistication ranging up to miniature catheter-tipped manometers are now readily available. The great advantage of all these systems is that their physical characteristics are fully understood so that the accuracy of each measurement can be checked, thereby increasing the validity of interpretation. Furthermore, they are very sensitive and respond to all pressure pulses, so that beat-by-beat pressures rather than 15-beat estimates are possible. However, the direct method does not measure exactly the same thing as the indirect method. The cannula faces upstream and therefore measures the forces at the leading edge of the pressure wave rather than the lateral forces on the wall of the artery.

EVALUATION OF THE INDIRECT METHOD

The contrast between the direct and indirect methods of measuring blood pressure has attracted much attention over the years. Because the direct method has obvious advantages of sensitivity and accuracy, it has been adopted as the "gold standard" against which to judge the indirect method. The first comparison of this kind was performed by Wolf and Von Bonsdorff in 1931 (37) and there have been many such comparisons since (30).

In all of these published comparisons, it is assumed that the direct technique is providing a "gold standard" by which the indirect technique must be judged. This cannot be justified, because the indirect technique is attempting to measure the lateral forces on the wall of the brachial artery, whereas the direct technique is measuring forces at the leading edge of the pressure wave moving down the column of blood in the artery. The two are bound to be similar, but could hardly be expected to be the same. Thus, the consistent demonstration of a high degree of correlation should cause no surprise, but there should be a systematic difference between the two sets of results. This is rendered unlikely by the use of one arm for the direct, and the other for the indirect, measurement. Furthermore, most workers appear to assume that the direct technique is perfect, and take no account of phenomena such as phase shift, which can significantly distort the direct measurements; hence, the almost universal failure to publish details of the physical characteristics of the apparatus used for direct measurements.

Only one published study has compared the two techniques in the same arm at the same time, and also gave details of the frequency characteristics of the direct apparatus to justify the accuracy of the method (30). This study was performed in females of a limited age range only, but is still the only study in which comparisons were made under ideal conditions for both methods. The results (Fig. 1) showed the expected close correlation between the two methods, but also showed considerable individual deviations that appeared to be random and were certainly not systematic. The fact that systolic pressure may deviate by as much as ± 24 mmHg and diastolic pressure by ± 16 mmHg under ideal conditions must provoke thought about the intrinsic accuracy of the indirect method.

The list of possible reasons for these random discrepancies is very impressive:

1. *Cuff*. Five features of the bladder design and application are known to produce errors. First, the evidence suggests that the best results are obtained if the bladder completely encircles the arm (14), and yet this is never the case with commercially available equipment. Second, failure to ensure that the bladder is placed over the artery can render a measurement completely invalid. Third, the width of the bladder is standardized at 12 cm, whereas the evidence suggests that the width should vary with the arm diameter (× 1.2 cm). Fourth, the fit of the cuff is essential if pressure is to be transmitted uniformly to the subcutaneous tissues (31). Finally, the shape of the cuff can be critical, particularly in obese subjects (21).
2. *Manometer*. The rates of inflation and deflation are known to effect the readings obtained. The recommended deflation rate of 2 to 3 mmHg/sec is seldom observed with any accuracy. Then there are the problems of observer bias and digit preference (6), which may well introduce further errors. Finally, servicing of the equipment is a vital factor—dirt in the inflation bulb or in the mercury can further compound an error.
3. *Auscultation*. Although it is generally agreed that the first appearance of sound (Korotkoff I) gives a good estimate of systolic pressure, there is still no definitive evidence on the correct auscultatory point for diastolic pressure. On physiological grounds, muffling (Korotkoff IV) should be the best point, but direct comparison suggests that disappearance (Korotkoff V) correlates better with direct diastolic pressure (30). It is also easier to detect than muffling, and hence it is universally recommended as the diastolic point. But this begs the question of the 5% of individuals who have marked silent intervals, or sounds that persist down to zero pressure. The unpredictability of these phenomena is bound to introduce further discrepancies.
4. *The artery*. It is well known that there may be differences between the two arms, and although this can be avoided by always using the right arm, it is still a possible source of error. Arteriosclerotic changes in the wall of the artery quite certainly influ-

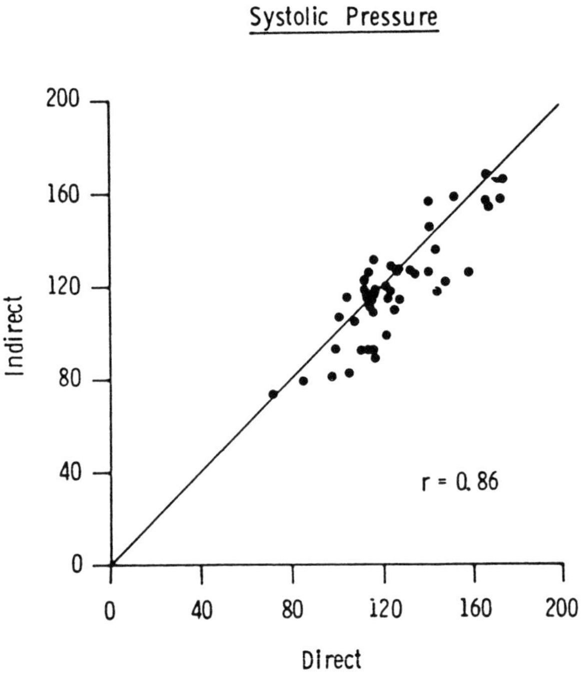

A

FIG. 1. A,B,C: Direct comparisons of direct and indirect (London School of Hygiene and Tropical Medicine instrument) blood pressure taken in the same arm at the same time under ideal measuring conditions. Note that the indirect technique can be at variance from the direct in individuals by as much as ±24/16 mmHg. The reasons for this variation, which appears to be random, have yet to be explained. (Redrawn from ref. 30.)

ence the transmission of sound: hence the pseudohypertension described by Osler at the turn of the century (22).

How many other sources of error exist that have yet to be defined remains a problem. Whatever they may be, the indirect technique can only be described as potentially inaccurate, unreliable, and so slow-moving as to be limited in its reliability. Furthermore, the indirect technique may be rendered even more inaccurate by the "alerting reaction" vividly described by Pickering (27) and now given a variety of other names such as "white-coat" hypertension. This phenomenon is characterized by a smart rise in blood pressure at the approach of a doctor (Fig. 2). The indirect method is incapable of detecting or quantifying the alerting reaction, which has been

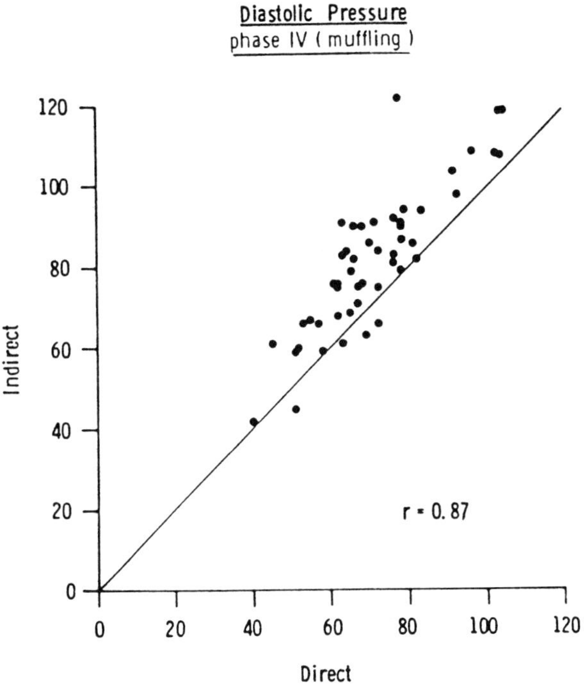
Diastolic Pressure
phase IV (muffling)
120
100
80
60
40
20
0
Indirect
r = 0.87
0
20
40
60
80
100
120
Direct

B

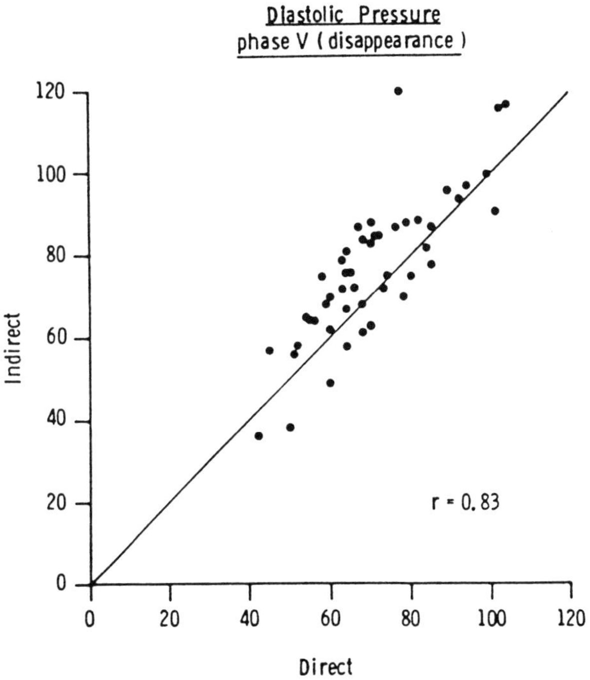
Diastolic Pressure
phase V (disappearance)
120
100
80
60
40
20
0
Indirect
r = 0.83
0
20
40
60
80
100
120
Direct

C

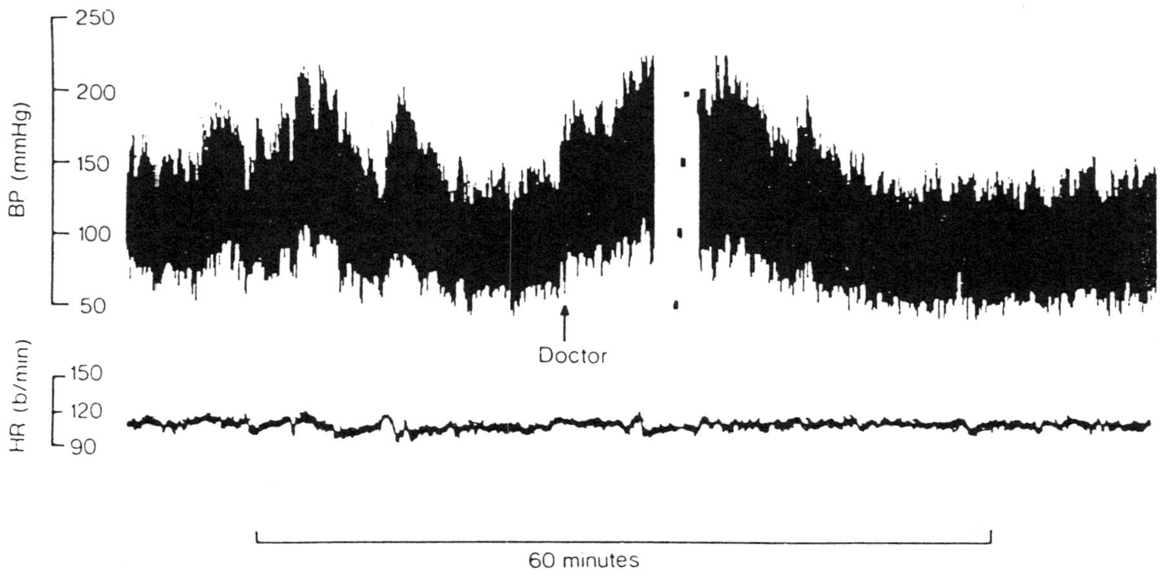

FIG. 2. A direct recording of the response of blood pressure to the presence of a physician in a hospitalized subject. The physician was well known to the patient, who was fully acquainted with the procedure. Note the absence of tachycardia in this pronounced "alerting reaction."

elegantly demonstrated by the direct technique. It has been shown that nurses elicit a smaller rise in pressure than doctors (17), but it is not possible to predict which subject will react in this way or the degree of the reaction.

MULTIPLE MEASUREMENTS

Physicians have long been aware of the drawbacks inherent in the Riva-Rocci/Korotkoff technique and the possibility of inaccurate recordings leading to wrong decisions. The clinician is more interested in the prognostic power of a reading than in its precision, but the indirect technique is so imprecise that it hardly inspires confidence. This was clearly illustrated by the work of Goldberg (7), who showed that clinic readings of blood pressure in treated hypertensive patients could be grossly misleading and might lead to increasing dosage of antihypertensive drugs to levels that could be dangerous (Fig. 3). He also drew attention to the fact that conclusions about the efficacy of antihypertensive therapy drawn from clinical trials using the indirect method could also be very misleading.

On the other hand, repeated measurements would seem to be more likely to provide a representative value and have a powerful appeal for the practicing physician (29). Most authorities (23) recommend that readings should be repeated at regular intervals on at least three occasions before any decisions are taken, despite the lack of evidence that such a mean level contains any more (or less) prognostic information than a single casual reading.

Another approach to the same problem is typified by the work of Smirk and his coworkers (1). They measured the blood pressure repeatedly under conditions of sedation and sensory deprivation and defined the lowest reading obtained in any one individual as the basal blood pressure. The difference between this and the casual reading was defined as the supplemental blood pressure. They produced evidence (33) that the basal blood pressure contained more prognostic information than the supplemental, thereby introducing the idea that the time of day might have a significance in determining both the level and the prognostic importance of a blood pressure reading.

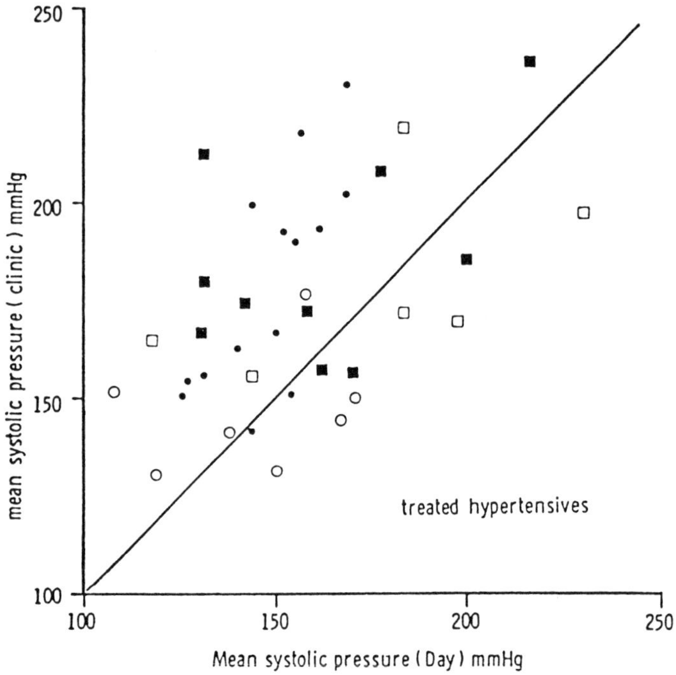
250
200
150
100
100
150
200
250
mean systolic pressure (clinic) mmHg
Mean systolic pressure (Day) mmHg
treated hypertensives

A

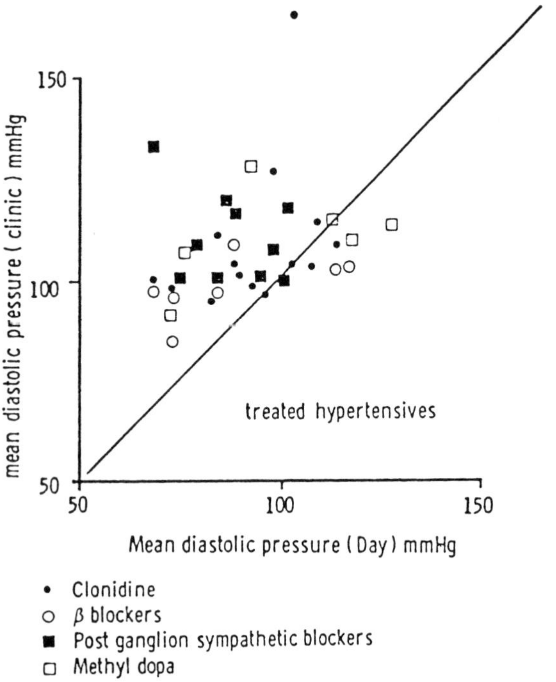
150
100
50
50
100
150
mean diastolic pressure (clinic) mmHg
Mean diastolic pressure (Day) mmHg
treated hypertensives
• Clonidine
○ β blockers
■ Post ganglion sympathetic blockers
□ Methyl dopa

B

AMBULATORY RECORDING

If multiple recordings are likely to improve precision and give more useful clinical information, then it is only logical to train patients to record their own blood pressure using the indirect technique and thereby obtain the required number of readings. This approach has been attempted by a number of physicians (5), but suffers from the lack of recordings during sleep.

The most significant advance in this direction came with the development of indirect ambulatory blood pressure recording by Sokolow and his coworkers (13) in San Francisco. They developed a portable recorder that utilized a microphone over the brachial artery and a manual inflate/deflate mechanism for a cuff around the arm. The Remler semiautomatic machine is the direct linear descendant of the Sokolow instrument, and has been supplemented by many others, such as the Avionics and the Squibb instruments. In fact new semiautomatic instruments are appearing on the market at a rate of about 10 per year.

Using the semiautomatic instrument, Sokolow and his coworkers (26) produced evidence that the ambulatory blood pressure was a better predictor of target organ damage that the casual clinic blood pressure. It is noteworthy that they also found ambulatory and office pressures to be equal as predictors of future events; by the time they made this observation it was clear that active intervention could be effective in reducing the incidence of cardiovascular complications of hypertension, and it was no longer ethically reasonable to withhold treatment in order to test a scientific hypothesis. For this reason it is not likely that the predictive superiority of ambulatory blood pressure, if it exists, will ever be clearly demonstrated.

It is surprising that the Sokolow experiment produced the result that it did. All the available indirect ambulatory techniques use the same basic principles as the Riva-Rocci/Korotkoff technique and must be open to the same inaccuracies. Furthermore, all indirect techniques involve the cessation of physical and mental activity dur-

FIG. 3. A,B: Relationship between clinic blood pressure (mean of three) and mean intra-arterial daytime blood pressure in treated hypertensives. The clinic readings are higher than the intra-arterial, a fact that might lead to unnecessary increases in dosage of medication. (Redrawn from ref. 7.)

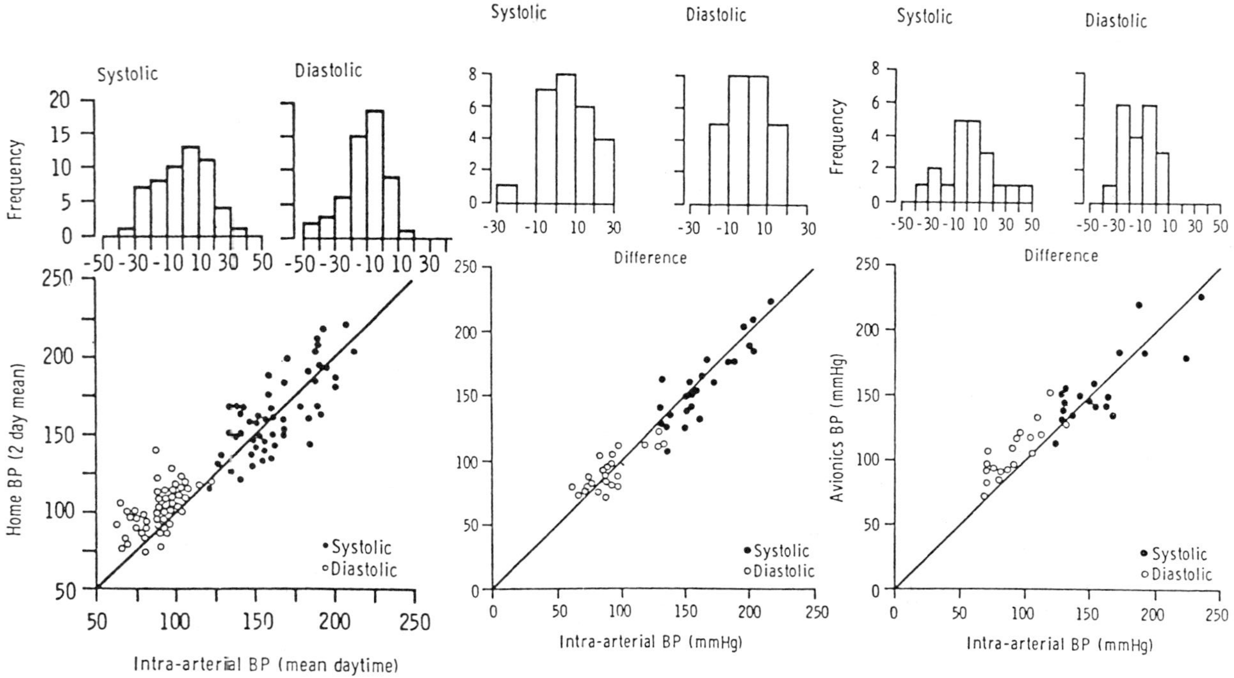

FIG. 4. Scatter plots and histograms comparing intra-arterial daytime blood pressure with home-recorded (anaeroid) and the Remler 2000 and Avionics Pressurometer II semiautomatic machines. The line of identity is drawn for each comparison and the incidence histograms give the difference frequencies. The scatter is greater for the home blood pressure, but the frequency histograms are very similar.

ing recording, and seldom give an accurate measurement of blood pressure during sleep.

Careful independent evaluations (8,11) have shown that the Remler and Avionics systems produce the same results as home self-recorded blood pressures using an anaeroid manometer (Fig. 4). Furthermore (9,10), they are no better at replicating the results of continuous intra-arterial recordings, and may show some potentially serious deviations in directional movement over time (Fig. 5). Despite the plethora of noninvasive reports, the unhappy truth is that these noninvasive ambulatory techniques have lagged behind the invasive methods in precision and accuracy of results, and are likely to do so until such time as the Riva-Rocci/Korotkoff principle can be replaced by another technique that will come closer in accuracy and sensitivity to the direct method. In the meantime, the conclu-

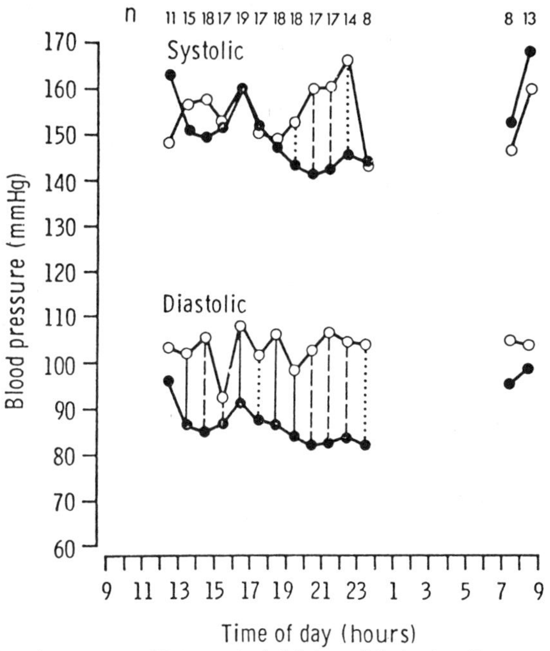

FIG. 5. Hourly means of intra-arterial (●) and Avionics Pressurometer II (○) blood pressure. The semiautomatic machine overreads for diastolic pressure, and there is a marked deviation in the direction of trend for systolic pressure.

sion of Gould (8) that these instruments give reasonable results when applied to *groups* of patients but do not when applied to individual patients must be borne in mind when interpreting results.

DIRECT INTRA-ARTERIAL RECORDINGS

The invasive nature of the direct technique has precluded widespread application in clinical studies of blood pressure; hence, the significance of the method for direct ambulatory blood pressure recording developed by Stott and his coworkers (2) in the laboratories of Sir George Pickering at Oxford University in the 1960s. This technique is essentially a research tool, but has provided powerful pathophysiological information on blood pressure that was never previously available. Many studies have outlined the way in which blood pressure responds to the activities of daily life (16,35), but the most important observations have stemmed from the application of statistical methods to the plethora of data obtained from such studies.

The application of coherent averaging to hourly means of systolic and diastolic blood pressure and heart rate in normal and hypertensive subjects has confirmed the presence of a long-suspected circadian rhythm of blood pressure, with highest readings in the morning and the lowest during the night (Fig. 6) (24). The only significant difference between the hypertensive and normal groups was a relative failure of the blood pressure to fall at night. Crucial to this description was the finding of a slow rise in pressure between the nadir at 3 AM and the rapid rise around the hour of awakening. Regrouping the data around the documented hour of awakening confirmed that this slow rise is a true event, and draws a sharp distinction between the behavior of blood pressure and heart rate, which continues to fall throughout this time. Further observations

FIG. 6. Circadian variation of blood pressure and heart rate in normotensive and hypertensive subjects, displayed by the technique of coherent averaging of hourly means. There are two peaks of blood pressure during the day and a steady rise before the hour of awakening. By way of contrast, heart rate peaks once, at a different time, and does not change until the time of awakening.

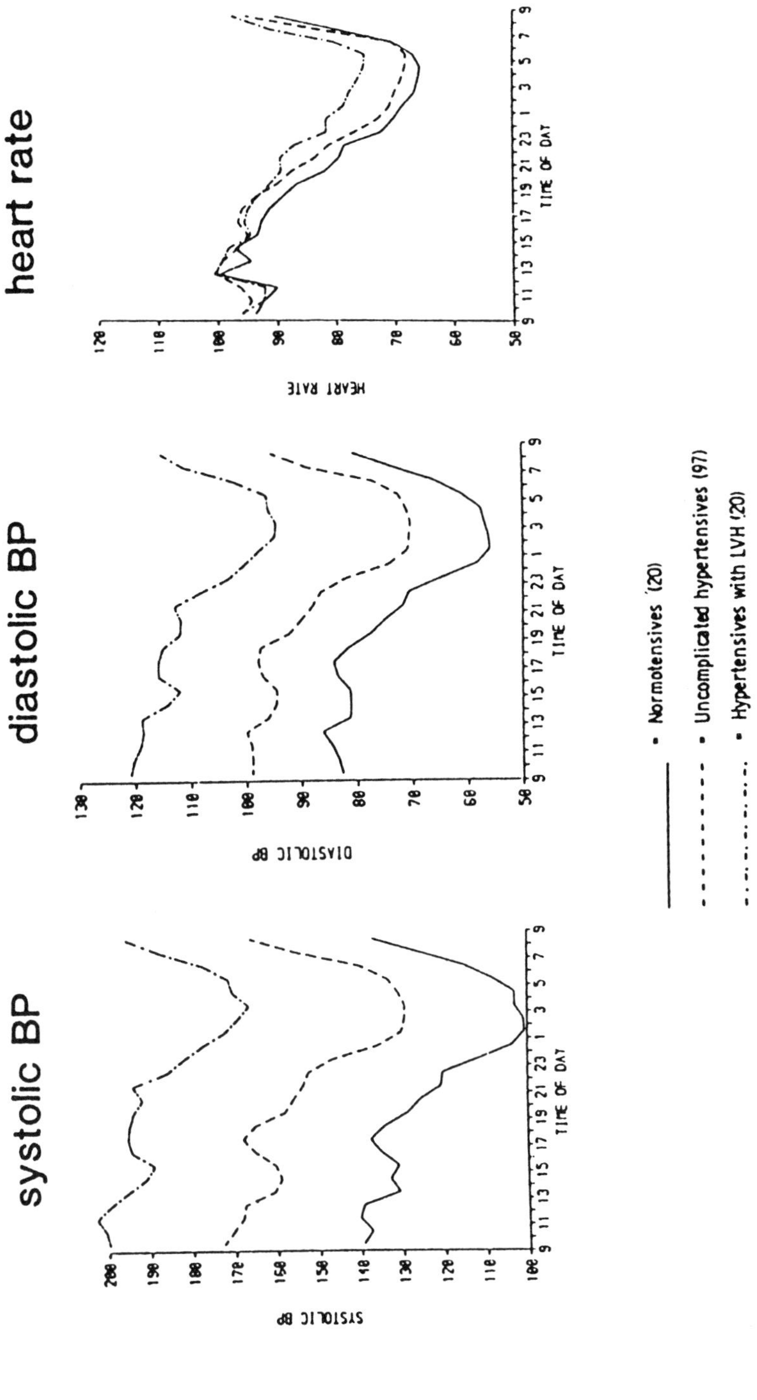
heart rate
diastolic BP
systolic BP
HEART RATE
DIASTOLIC BP
SYSTOLIC BP
TIME OF DAY
Normotensives (20)
Uncomplicated hypertensives (97)
Hypertensives with LVH (20)

have confirmed that this rhythm of blood pressure is not a simple alternation of activity and inactivity (19), and recordings in patients with fixed-rate pacemakers (4) have confirmed the divergence in behavior of blood pressure and heart rate. These observations fit well with other evidence (15) of increased sympathetic activity during the morning and have focused attention upon the possibility that blood pressure may be reflecting a series of physiological events that might be responsible for the increased incidence of stroke (3) and myocardial infarction (25) at this time of day.

This conclusion was supported by the finding that central and peripheral sympathetic denervation produces a reversal of the rhythm, with highest pressures during the night and lowest during the day (18). This suggests that the sympathetic nervous system is imposing a rhythm upon the body that is a complete reversal of what would otherwise happen. The same effect has been reported in patients after heart transplant (34), which raises the interesting possibility that the drive for this sympathetic activity may be originating in the heart itself.

This rhythm has been shown to be highly reproducible, both in the short- and long-term in groups of hypertensive subjects, and is not subject to a placebo effect (12). This makes this approach particularly suitable for clinical trials of antihypertensive drugs.

WHICH BLOOD PRESSURE?

For the practicing clinician, the question of prognosis still remains the most important issue in deciding the correct management for an individual patient. Although blood pressure alone is not the only factor to be considered in assessing the risk of cardiovascular disease, at the end of the day this measurement is still a powerful and independent predictor. Furthermore, it would appear that the number and the timing of recordings may increase predictive accuracy. A recent study (20) of the predictive accuracy of casual and 24-hour intra-arterial blood pressure recordings for target organ damage and cardiovascular events over a 5-year period has confirmed the power of casual blood pressure readings, but has also shown that the 24-hour mean blood pressure increases this power dramatically (Fig. 7). Most of this predictive power resides in the mean pressures between midnight and noon. This data supports the work of Smirk in stressing the importance of nocturnal blood pressure and must provide a powerful stimulus to the efforts to produce a method of accurately recording blood pressure at this time of the day.

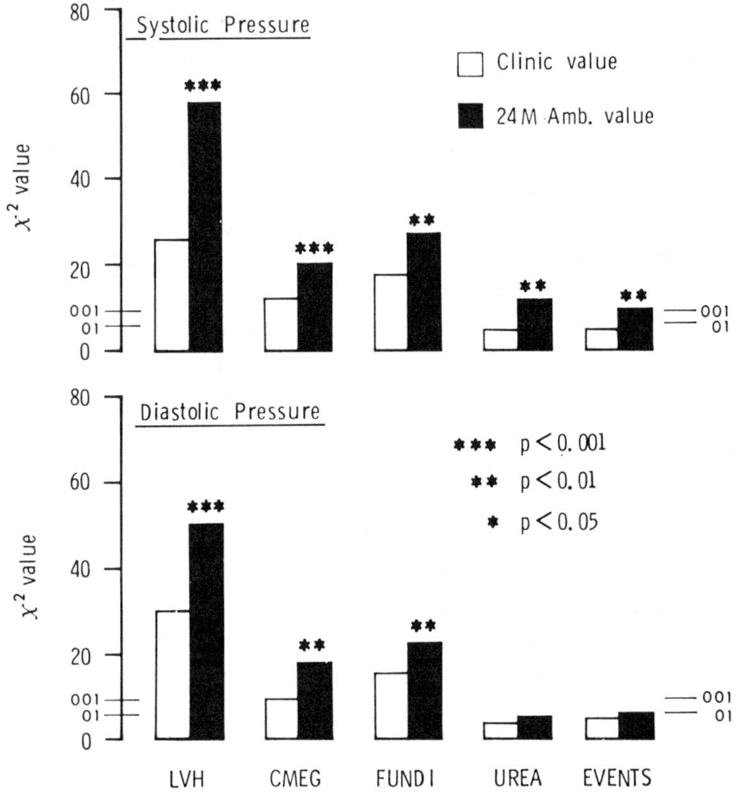

FIG. 7. The predictive value of the casual and 24-hr intra-arterial blood pressure for target organ damage and morbid events. Note the power of the casual blood pressure, but the much greater power of the intra-arterial 24-hr mean pressure. LVH, left ventricular hypertrophy; CMEG, cardiomegaly (x-ray); FUND 1, Grade II or more hyptensive fundal changes; UREA, raised blood urea; EVENTS, cardio-vascular events in a 5-year period.

CONCLUSIONS

The casual indirect blood pressure with all its drawbacks has undoubted power for the prediction of morbid cardiovascular events in populations, but there is considerable doubt about its value when applied to individuals. These doubts center upon the known inherent inaccuracies of the technique and the feeling that the sample is not big enough to be "representative." There are indications that repeated ambulatory measurements give better prognostic information in individuals, but all the indirect methods of recording that have been described to date suffer from the inherent inaccuracies of the Riva-Rocci/Korotkoff technique. The only accurate method available is the Oxford technique for ambulatory intra-arterial blood pressure recording. This has been successfully applied to normal and hypertensive subjects to describe the circadian rhythm of blood pressure and the changes produced by disease states. This rhythm is now widely used to assess the efficacy of antihypertensive drugs. Long-term studies are emphasizing the importance of nocturnal and morning blood pressure in the pathogenesis of cardiovascular disease states. The technique has also been applied to studies of angina and silent myocardial ischemia, which have highlighted the differences between ischemia induced by exercise and that which occurs "spontaneously" in a natural environment. Studies in heart failure have produced evidence that points to the heart as a central regulating organ in the circulation and not just a pump that responds to outside controlling influences. Despite the considerable contribution that the direct technique has made, it remains a research tool for application in only a few centers and strictly controlled conditions. The search for an equally accurate indirect method has not been very fruitful, but must go forward, since the need for such a technique is self-evident.

REFERENCES

1. Alam GM, Smirk FH. Casual and basal blood pressure in British and Egyptian Men. *Br Heart J* 1943;5:152–155.
2. Bevan AT, Honour AJ, Stott FM. Direct arterial blood pressure recording in unrestricted man. *Clin Sci* 1969;36:329–344.

3. Bock KD, Kreuzenbeck W. Spontaneous blood pressure variations in hypertension: the effect of anti-hypertensive therapy and correlations with the incidence of complications. In: Gross F, ed. *Anti-hypertensive therapy. Principles and practice*. Berlin: Springer, 1966;224–228.
4. Davies AB, Gould BA, Cashman PMM, Raftery EB. Circadian rhythm of blood pressure in patients dependent on ventricular demand pacemakers. *Br Heart J* 1984;52:93–98.
5. Editorial. Self measurement of blood pressure. *Lancet* 1985;2:377–378.
6. Eilertsen E., Humerfelt S. The observer variation in the measurement of arterial blood pressure. *Acta Med Scand* 1968;184:145–157.
7. Goldberg AD. Blood pressure and heart rate in ambulant hypertensives. MD Thesis, University of Sheffield, 1976.
8. Gould BA. An evaluation of indirect methods of ambulatory blood pressure recording. MD Thesis, University of London, 1982.
9. Gould BA, Hornung RS, Cashman PMM, Altman D, Raftery EB. An evaluation of the Avionics Pressurometer III 1978 at home and in hospital. *Clin Cardiol* 1986;9:335–343.
10. Gould BA, Hornung RS, Kieso HA, Altman DG, Cashman PMM, Raftery EB. Evaluation of the Remler M2000 Blood Pressure Recorder. *Hypertension* 1984;6:209–215.
11. Gould BA, Hornung RS, Kieso H, Cashman PMM, Raftery EB. An evaluation of home-recorded blood pressure during trials. *Hypertension* 1986;8:267–271.
12. Gould BA, Mann S, Davies AB, Altman DG, Raftery EB. Does placebo lower blood pressure? *Lancet* 1981;2:1377–1381.
13. Kain H, Hinman AT, Sokolow M. Arterial blood pressure measurements with a portable blood pressure recorder in hypertensive patients. *Circulation* 1964;30:882–892.
14. King GE. Some sources of error in the clinical measurement of blood pressure. MD Thesis, University of London, 1967.
15. Linsell CR, Lightman SL, Mullen PE, Brown MJ, Causon RC. Circadian rhythms of epinephrine and nor-epinephrine in man. *J Clin Endocrinol Metab* 1985;60:1210–1215.
16. Littler WA, Honour AJ, Sleight P. Direct arterial pressure, pulse rate, and electrocardiogram during micturition and defecation in unrestricted man. *Am Heart J* 1974;88:205–210.
17. Mancia G, Bertinieri G, Grassi G, Parati G, Pomidossi G, Ferrai A, Gregorini L, Zanchetti A. Effects of blood pressure measurement by the doctor on patient's blood pressure and heart rate. *Lancet* 1983;2:695–698.
18. Mann S, Altman D, Raftery EB, Bannister R. Circadian variation of blood pressure in autonomic failure. *Circulation* 1983;68:477–483.
19. Mann S, Miller Craig MW, Melville D, BalaSubramanian V, Raftery EB. Physical activity and the circadian rhythm of blood pressure. *Clin Sci* 1979;57(Suppl 5):375s–377s.
20. Mann S, Miller Craig MW, Raftery EB. Superiority of 24 hour measurement of blood pressure over clinic values in determining prognosis in hypertension. *Clin Exp Hypertens* 1985;7:279–281.
21. Maxwell GF, Pruijt JFM, Arntzenuis DC. Comparison of the conical cuff and the standard rectangular cuffs. *Int J Epidemiol* 1985;14:468–472.

22. Messerli FH, Ventura HO, Amodeo C. Osler's maneuver and pseudohypertension. *New Engl J Med* 1985;312:1548–1551.
23. Miall WE. Screening for hypertension. *Br J Hosp Med* 1982;592–594.
24. Miller Craig MW, Bishop CN, Raftery EB. Circadian variation of blood. *Lancet* 1978;1:795–797.
25. Myers A, Dewar HA. Circumstances attending 100 sudden deaths from coronary artery disease with Coroners Necropsies. *Br Heart J* 1975;37:1133–1143.
26. Perloff D, Sokolow M, Cowan R. The prognostic value of ambulatory blood pressures. *JAMA* 1983;249:2792–2798.
27. Pickering GW. *High blood pressure*. London: J & A Churchill, 1974;15–17.
28. Raftery EB. The methodology of blood pressure recording. *Br J Clin Pharmacol* 1978;6:193–198.
29. Raftery EB. Hypertension: Who and when to treat. *Update* 1985;155–158.
30. Raftery EB, Ward AP. The indirect method of recording blood pressure. *Cardiovasc Res* 1968;2:210–218.
31. Rushmer RF. *Cardiovascular dynamics*. Philadelphia and London: WB Saunders, 1961;137.
32. Sigerist, HE *A history of medicine*, vol 1. England, *Oxford University Press*, 1955;311,329.
33. Smirk FH. Observations on the mortality of 270 treated and 199 untreated grade 1 and 2 hypertensive patients followed in all instances for 5 years. *N Z Med J* 1964;63:413–443.
34. Wenting GJ, Meiracker AH, Eck HJ, Simoons ML, Bos E, Weimar W, ManIn't Veld AJ, Schalekamp MADH. Lack of circadian variation of blood pressure after heart transplant. *J Hypertens* 1986;4(Suppl 6):578–580.
35. Wertheimer L, Bandul I, Amarasinghe S. *Blood pressure in normal subjects. Second International Symposium on Ambulatory Monitoring*. London: Academic Press, 1977;143–148.
36. Wiggers CJ, ed. *Physiology in health and disease*. Philadelphia: Lea & Febiger, 1934;604–608.
37. Wolf HT, Von Bonsdorff B. Blutige messung der absoluten Sphygmogramms beim Menschen. *Z Gesamte Exper Med* 1931;79:569–577.

Ambulatory Blood Pressure Recording,
edited by H. Brunner and B. Waeber.
Raven Press, Ltd., New York © 1992.

3

Ambulatory Blood Pressure and Assessment of Cardiovascular Risk

*Dorothee Perloff and †Maurice Sokolow

**Division of Cardiology, Department of Medicine, and †Department of Medicine and Cardiovascular Research Institute, University of California at San Francisco, San Francisco, California 94143*

Hypertension is a prevalent chronic disease in all Western countries, and inappropriate high blood pressure results in cardiac hypertrophy, and acceleration of artherosclerosis in both the muscular conduit arteries and the smaller resistance arteries and arterioles. Consequently hypertension is one of the major precursors of premature death and morbidity from congestive heart failure, and ischemic cardiac, cerebral, peripheral vascular, and renal disease (25,58,101, 103). The lowest level of blood pressure that warrants a diagnosis of hypertension is arbitrary and controversial, and it is questionable whether all individuals with mild blood pressure elevation are equally at risk (61,92). There is no debate, however, that the higher the blood pressure level, the greater is the likelihood that the individual will eventually develop clinical hypertension and involvement of target organs, and, ultimately, clinical cardiovascular complications (33,46,64,65). The progressive increase in morbidity in groups of individuals with increasingly higher levels of blood pressure has been well documented by large insurance companies as well as by epidemiologic studies on normal and hypertensive populations (14,109,112).

Yet the *level of blood pressure* is an ill-defined term for describing a physiologic variable that fluctuates widely with sleep and arousal, day and night, work and play, exercise and rest, stress and anger, eating and other bodily functions (61,92). Which level is it that is most predictive of outcome, most closely related to the extent of involvement of target organs? Is it the lowest pressure recorded after a period of rest or during sleep, is it the peak elevation that occurs with mental or physical arousal, is it the variability or the range of the fluctuations, or is it an average of all the pressures throughout the 24 hours?

UNRELIABILITY OF OFFICE PRESSURE

In large epidemiologic studies the blood pressure is usually determined on several visits or screenings before individuals are labeled hypertensive and stratified into treatment groups. Several investigators have shown that three readings are more predictive of the subsequent level of the blood pressure than one reading, and measurements made on multiple occasions are more reliable than multiple measurements made on one occasion (4,5,12,74). In the Hypertension Detection and Follow-up Program, 40% of the individuals who had a diastolic pressure above 95 mmHg on the initial house-to-house screening, had a pressure less than 90 mmHg on a subsequent examination (51). In the Australian National High Blood Pressure Study, 48% of the placebo-treated hypertensive patients had a fall in pressure from an initial level above 95 mmHg to below 95 mmHg after 3 years of observation, making it questionable that the initial diagnosis of hypertension was correct (6). In the Veterans Administration study, patients were hospitalized for several days and the lowest pressure on days 4 to 6 in the hospital plus the pressures after 2 weeks of outpatient observation were used for classification before randomization into treatment groups (30). Many investigators have described a progressive fall of the blood pressure, often to normal levels, in hospitalized patients (50,77,79).

Thus, it is widely recognized that a single initial blood pressure recorded in the doctor's office can differ considerably from subsequent measurements made after several office visits and from repeated measurements made at home by the patient or a relative. Any one measurement is not necessarily representative of the blood pressure levels during the entire 24 hr. There are several explanations for these observations in addition to the concept of "regression toward the mean." One is the normal variability of blood pressure, the fluctuation in level corresponding to the circadian rhythm of the blood pressure and the varying states of physiologic arousal. The second is the role of familiarity with the medical environment, the degree of sensitization to the physician, the activation of the "fight-flight" reaction, so aptly described by Sir George Pickering (91).

THE VARIABILITY OF BLOOD PRESSURE

The fluctuation of the arterial blood pressure during 24 hr and from one measurement to the next is well recognized. Armitage and Rose (5) described a study in which they obtained duplicate readings on each of 20 occasions on 10 subjects, using bias-free standardized techniques and equipment. The within-subject variability ranged from 25 to 30 mmHg, and the between-occasion variation was as much as a 12 mmHg fall for diastolic pressure between the first and the 20th occasion. They inferred that the precision of any study of blood pressure would be improved by taking multiple measurements. Furthermore they recommended that although it is easier to obtain multiple measurements on the same occasion, the precision of the measurement would be improved if the readings were obtained on different occasions. Subsequently, Armitage and coworkers (4) studied the variability of measurements of casual blood pressure in a group of 722 men who had been examined annually for 4 successive years. The standard deviation, representing the random difference between occasions for individual subjects, was estimated to be 9.1 mmHg for systolic and 7.2 mmHg for diastolic pressure. If a label of hypertension had been attached on the basis of a single reading, the prevalence of hypertension in this group would have been overestimated by at least 17%.

Glock and coworkers (36) obtained six resting blood pressure measurements at 5-min intervals, daily at the same time of day, for 3 weeks in one group of 21 subjects. In another group of 15 subjects they obtained measurements three times daily: morning, noon, and night. They found that no single reading or group of readings obtained on a single day could serve as an index of the variability of the blood pressure over the 3-week period of the study. Similar investigations have been reported by other observers, and the consensus is that any epidemiologic or treatment study must incorporate a measure of blood pressure variability (37,105,116).

The mechanism of the fluctuation of the blood pressure, and the circadian rhythms of many other physiologic variables is a subject of much current research, but such a discussion is beyond the scope of this chapter (11,16,27,66,78,122).

THE FIGHT-FLIGHT REACTION

In addition to the inherent variability of the blood pressure from measurement to measurement, another factor contributes to the unreliability of measurements made at any one time in the physician's office. Many patients react to having their blood pressure measured with a conscious or unconscious alarm reaction, the "orienting" or "defense" reaction (91,95). This response consists of a rise in the blood pressure and heart rate which teleologically prepares the "animal" for a response such as flight from or fight with the adversary, here, the physician. Other features of this reaction include vasoconstriction in the skin and intestines and dilatation of the pupils. This reaction can be partially extinguished by repetitive measurements over time. Sir George Pickering and coworkers (93) described the progressive drop in pressure from 200/110 mmHg to 150/100 mmHg over a 12-week period in a patient whose pressure was measured weekly in the clinic while he was receiving a placebo. In a recent study of 292 patients with borderline or mild hypertension who were studied with ambulatory pressure recordings, T. G. Pickering and coworkers (95) found that 21% had normal blood pressures during the day. These patients were considered to have only "white-coat" hypertension, rather than sustained hypertension (95).

The fall in blood pressure that is observed in hospitalized patients may also represent a desensitization to the medical environment and to having the blood pressure measured, as well as a removal from a stressful work environment. Mancia and coworkers (71), using a continuous intra-arterial blood pressure monitoring device in hospitalized patients, reported that in some the systolic blood pressure rose 30 mmHg and the diastolic 20 mmHg when a physician entered the room. The peak rise occurred within 2 to 4 min after the physician entered. In some patients the height of the rise was not diminished with subsequent visits by the doctor over a 2-day period. Of interest is that the blood pressure also rose, but less so, when a nurse entered the room.

BASAL BLOOD PRESSURES

Addis (1), and later Alam and Smirk (2), observed that measurements made on individuals at rest and in a basal state were lower than measurements made casually during a busy day, and were more reproducible. Smirk and coworkers (108) popularized the use of "basal" blood pressure determinations, both for making a diagnosis of hypertension and predicting outcome, and for assessing the effects of drug therapy. They differentiated between the "basal" and the "supplemental pressure," defined as the difference between the casual and the basal pressures. In a prospective epidemiologic study Smirk observed that the 8-year cumulative mortality among 245 hypertensive patients was positively correlated with the basal blood pressure, but did not correlate with the "supplemental" pressure (107). On the basis of these observations Smirk recommended the use of the basal blood pressure as a reliable and reproducible measurement of a patient's blood pressure, which correlated well with both severity and prognosis.

HOME BLOOD PRESSURES

Another method for obtaining more representative and reproducible measurements of blood pressure is to measure the blood pressures while the patient is at home (127). The patient measures the blood pressure on himself with an appropriate self-adjustable cuff with a built-in stethoscope. Alternatively, a nonthreatening relative can measure the blood pressure. Most patients can be taught to measure their pressure with reasonable accuracy. Many machines are now available for this purpose which automatically record the pressure and provide a digital display of the numbers without the need for the patient to listen for the Korotkoff sounds. Unfortunately none of these is reliably and reproducibly accurate, and regular calibration and maintenance of such equipment remains a problem (80,81).

Ayman and Goldshine (7) reported that home blood pressure measurements were lower than office pressures in their patients, and could be used as a reliable guide to the effectiveness of antihypertensive therapy. They found that the highest pressure obtained at home was as much as 50 mmHg lower than the highest reading obtained in the physician's office. The lowest readings were those taken after a 20-min rest in the office or at the end of each session at home. In several of their patients with malignant hypertension there was very little difference between the office and the home pressures, both were high, and these patients died early. Other patients with high office pressures but low pressures at home, lived for many years without major complications. Ayman and Goldshine suggested that home pressures correlated better with outcome than did office pressures, and, additionally, could be used to make patients less fearful of their condition and more compliant with therapy (7).

Freis (29) made a similar observation in 32 patients treated with ganglion-blocking drugs whose home blood pressures suggested effective blood pressure control in all but one patient, whereas the office pressures remained elevated in two-thirds of the patients. If the patients who were well controlled at home had been treated according to their office pressures, they would have been overtreated, and unnecessarily subjected to the unpleasant side effects of the potent ganglion-blocking drugs. Ibrahim and coworkers (52) also observed that the effectiveness of therapy in reducing the degree of left ventricular hypertrophy, as measured by the electrocardiogram, correlated better with home pressures than with office pressures. Padfield and coworkers (82) suggested that the measurements made at home predicted the office pressure on the third visit, and therefore could be used as a substitute for making measurements on repeated office visits. Other investigators have made similar observations and home blood pressure measurements have been used in several large-scale drug treatment trials (42,56,80).

HISTORY OF AMBULATORY BLOOD PRESSURE MONITORING

In 1961, we observed in a 5-year prognostic study of 439 hypertensive patients (112) that although the pressures obtained on the initial office visit, after a period of rest in a quiet room, were predictive of outcome in the majority of patients, there were patients with substantially raised pressures who showed no evidence of target organ abnormality and who survived for many years despite the high pressures obtained in the office. We theorized that some of these patients might have had transiently high pressures in the office that were not sustained and thus did not reflect the pressures during the remainder of the day. To evaluate the blood pressure away from the medical environment, Sokolow, with the technical assistance of Singer from the University of California at Berkeley, initiated the development of equipment for measuring and recording the blood pressure repeatedly in ambulatory patients. The preliminary results with the Remler portometer, which uses the occluding-cuff Korotkoff technique for measuring the pressure, were reported by Hinman et al. (47) in 1962. This apparatus, which records the blood pressures on a magnetic tape, enabled us to make repeated measurements away from the medical environment, and to sample blood pressure levels during various daytime activities. From these records we were able to determine an average or mean pressure for the whole day, which, we theorized, would be more characteristic of the individual's pressure load, than the average of multiple office pressures.

Early experience with the Remler apparatus, which, since it requires manual cuff inflation, permits sampling only of "awake" pressures, suggested that such an apparatus was acceptable to patients, that multiple blood pressures could indeed be obtained without major inconvenience, and that the pressure obtained with the recorder corresponded well with simultaneous measurements made by a trained observer using a conventional manometer (17,47). Other investigators have subsequently validated the accuracy of the Remler apparatus (41). Since these measurements were performed away from the medical environment, we could avoid the potential alarm reaction induced by the presence of a physician. However, when the physician visited the patient at home, the blood pressure was invariably higher at the end of the day, than in the period preceding the doctor's visit (115).

Later, Kain and coworkers (57), working in our laboratory, reported that in 62 individuals, both hypertensive and normotensive, the average portable or ambulatory pressure was 12.2/9.6 mmHg lower than the corresponding average office pressure. Although the ambulatory pressure was lower than the office pressure in the majority of patients, some patients had peaks during the day that were higher than those recorded in the office. These investigators confirmed the reproducibility of the ambulatory measurements on each of 3 successive days, and on repeated measurements made a month apart. In an occasional patient the pressures were higher on the first of the 3 days, presumably due to the novelty of wearing the recording apparatus, which subsequently wore off. They also observed that the highest pressures occurred in the morning, and that the pressure level progressively declined during the day, interrupted only by superimposed fluctuations related to changing activities and moods. For this group of patients the standard deviation did not correlate with the mean pressure for the whole day, and for each mean pressure there were wide fluctuations between the five highest readings and the five lowest readings.

Shortly thereafter several other investigators developed equipment for measuring blood pressures in ambulatory patients (99, 104). Richardson (99), working in Sir George Pickering's laboratory, initially used an oscillographic device with an automatic, self-inflating double pneumatic cuff, which made it possible to obtain readings both by day and at night. With this he confirmed the marked fall in blood pressure that occurs during sleep, as had previously been demonstrated in hospitalized patients. Subsequently the "Oxford technique" was developed by Bevan et al. (8), which involved the insertion of an intra-arterial catheter and which provided continuous beat-by-beat blood pressure information. With the help of computerization it became possible to average the pressures over any interval or time period, and to correlate the pressure levels with concurrent or simultaneous activities, rather than spacing the individual measurements at 20- to 30-min intervals. Continuous monitoring of intra-arterial pressure doubtless provides the most accurate information and the largest number of measurements, but is not widely acceptable because of the invasiveness of the technique and the limited number of studies that can be performed in an individual patient.

Using the Oxford technique, Littler and coworkers (67,68) and others (53,70,72,119,125) have made valuable observations relating daily events and activities to fluctuating blood pressure levels. This method has proved to be particularly useful for studying the variability of blood pressure, although similar observations have been made with indirect measurements and intermittent cuff inflation. More recently, a number of other automatic self-inflating devices have been developed, modified, and progressively perfected (15,24,49,69,76,94,96,106). These devices use the occluding cuff and Korotkoff sound technique, similar to the Remler, or the oscillometric method for measuring the blood pressure. With improvement in the devices they have become lighter, more streamlined, easier to apply, and the decoding of the blood pressure record has been computerized (43,48). Early results on the reproducibility of ambulatory measurements, the variability of the blood pressure and its circadian pattern, and the effect of environmental and emotional influences on the pressure have been validated and extended (24,54). However, standardization of the equipment, selection of the best techniques of measurement, identification of artifacts, and statistical management of the data remain subjects of discussion and controversy (81,117). Ambulatory blood pressure monitoring is still considered experimental by many health policy makers (45).

Several questions have been posed regarding ambulatory blood pressure monitoring. What is the optimum number of readings and the best interval between readings, and is it really necessary to monitor blood pressure for a full 24 hrs? What do the pressure recordings during sleep contribute (39)? Di Rienzo and coworkers (21,22) found that no single 1-hr or even 4-hr period gave the same information as the average derived from computerized beat-to-beat analysis of the entire continuous 24-hr recording. However, analysis of the averages of measurements made at 5-, 10-, 15-, and up to 30-min intervals during the 24 hr provided the same information as the 24-hr average derived from the continuous sample. The standard deviation obtained by analyzing the data only at 15-min intervals differed from the analysis obtained from the continuous 24-hr sample by only 10%. Parati and his group of investigators (84) also showed that the intermittent inflation of the cuff required for indirect measurement of the pressure did not produce a repeated alarm reaction when the pressure was simultaneously measured with a continuous intra-arterial device.

A major unanswered question remains: What is "normal" ambulatory blood pressure? Since the ambulatory pressure tends to be lower than the office pressure, the arbitrary dividing line between normal and abnormal, 140/90 mmHg, should perhaps not apply to ambulatory pressures. But how much lower should the dividing line be? The answer has major implications for the diagnosis of hypertension, for deciding whom to treat, and for determining when treatment is adequate or excessive (100,121,123,124). This question, What is the ambulatory pressure in normals?, has been addressed by several investigators who have compared the ambulatory pressures in small numbers of normal, borderline, and hypertensive individuals, mostly men, under various conditions (18,20,34,62,70,75,94, 98). All investigators have reported considerable overlap of individual ambulatory pressures among these groups, although the mean for the 24 hr is consistently higher in individuals labeled hypertensive. Only a few studies of blood pressure variability have been carried out in older individuals (24,63). The circadian pattern in normals resembles that observed in hypertensives, but peaks at a lower level. Likewise the blood pressure responses to various laboratory stresses have been studied in these groups, and, as expected, have shown exaggerated responses among borderline and hypertensive individuals (35,72). However, the reliability of all of the noninvasive blood pressure recorders at the height of exercise is limited (40). A large-scale study of normal individuals remains to be done. Such a study needs to include more women and individuals in all age ranges.

CORRELATION OF AMBULATORY PRESSURE WITH CARDIOVASCULAR COMPLICATIONS

The more or less linear relationship between the level of the office blood pressure and the severity or extent of involvement of the cardiovascular target organs has been described by many investigators (58,101,110). It is also recognized that the more advanced the degree of target organ involvement (such as left ventricular hypertrophy or changes in the optic fundi), the greater is the risk of the subsequent development of clinical cardiovascular complications and death (9,13,30,59,97,112). On the basis of experience with the Framingham cohort of 5,209 individuals who were initially free of cardiovascular disease, Kannel (58,60) found that the mean, maximum, and minimum of three blood pressures taken at one time were equally efficient predictors of cardiovascular disease. However, in a multivariate analysis, the risk of developing cardiovascular complications was unaffected by the degree of variability of the pressure, for any given average pressure.

Sokolow and Harris (110) reported that in a group of patients with essential hypertension who were largely untreated, 64% of those with an initial blood pressure less than 200/110 mmHg, had a normal electrocardiogram (ECG), and only 12% had advanced left ventricular hypertrophy (LVH). However, in the group with blood pressures above 250/130 mmHg (obtained in the office after a period of rest), 58% had advanced LVH and only 15% had a normal ECG. Among patients in the lower blood pressure group, only 5% had advanced changes in the optic fundi and over 50% had normal or near-normal eyegrounds, whereas in the higher blood pressure group, 37% had advanced funduscopic changes and only 7% had normal or near-normal eyegrounds. However, in this analysis there were some striking exceptions and inconsistencies: there were patients with high blood pressures in the office who had no target organ abnormalities and others with mild blood pressure elevation who had advanced LVH on the ECG (110).

Other investigators have also remarked on the disparity between the level of the blood pressure and left ventricular mass, as measured by echocardiography (23,32,52,126) and have speculated that the level of the pressure as measured in the office is not the sole determinant of hypertrophy, perhaps because it does not accurately represent the total pressure load on the left ventricle. The disparity between office blood pressure and the effect of antihypertensive therapy has already been alluded to (52). Taguchi and Freis (118), on reviewing the results of the Veterans Administration study, remarked that even those patients whose office diastolic pressure was not reduced below 90 mmHg had a considerable benefit from antihypertensive therapy.

It was appropriate, therefore, to investigate if ambulatory blood pressures correlated better with target organ damage than did office blood pressures. In a report on 124 individuals Sokolow and coworkers (114) related blood pressure level to degree of target organ damage or severity of hypertension. For each class of severity (based on abnormalities in the optic fundi, ECG, roentgenogram of the chest, and a measure of renal function), the average office and ambulatory blood pressures were progressively higher, but the average ambulatory pressure was consistently lower than the office pressure. Similarly for each higher degree of the specific measures of severity [ECG-LVH(111), radiologic cardiac size, optic fundi–KW classification (9)], the average pressure of patients so affected were higher. The investigators did not, however, find a relationship between variability (standard deviation of all ambulatory pressures) nor with duration of hypertension and severity (114).

Overall severity class correlated with both systolic and diastolic pressure, with both office and ambulatory pressure, but the correlation was better with ambulatory pressure, $r = .63$ for ambulatory systolic versus $r = .48$ for office systolic, and $r = .65$ for ambulatory diastolic versus $r = .51$ for office diastolic pressures (114). The correlation between severity and multiple variables combined was then analyzed by means of a stepwise multiple regression analysis. The degree of left ventricular hypertrophy by ECG correlated best with ambulatory systolic and diastolic pressure and age. Classification of the optic fundi correlated best with ambulatory systolic and diastolic pressure and age, although the addition of age to the analysis increased the degree of correlation only in those over age 45. Overall the correlation with severity was better for ambulatory than for office pressures. Thus ambulatory pressures explained 26% of the variance not accounted for by office blood pressures (114).

In attempting to define a level of ambulatory pressure above which target organ damage was prevalent and below which it was absent, Sokolow et al. (114) found that less that 1% of ambulatory diastolic pressures recorded in class I patients were greater than 110 mmHg, whereas 87% of diastolic pressures recorded in patients with class III to IV severity were in excess of 110 mmHg. Conversely, in class II patients, only 9% of diastolic readings were less than 80 mmHg, and in class III patients only 1% of readings were less than 90 mmHg. However, it must be remembered that a raised pressure is not only a risk factor for the development of target organ damage, but even in normotensives, the higher the pressure at any time, the greater is the risk of the subsequent development of clinical hypertension. Thus, Kooperstein et al. (64) reviewed the records of 652 employees of the Port Authority of New York who remained employed for 10 to 15 years. One percent of those who had a systolic pressure less than 140 mmHg on their preemployment physical examination subsequently developed clinical hypertension, whereas the incidence rose to 3.2% among those with an initial pressure of 140 to 149 mmHg and to 11.1% among those with initial pressures of 150 to 159 mmHg. Thus, even isolated office pressures may be predictive of outcome in groups of individuals.

Many observers have confirmed that ambulatory pressures correlate better with evidence of target organ damage than do the pressures obtained in the physician's office (10,19,31). Floras and coworkers (28) observed in a group of patients with essential hypertension who were studied with the Oxford technique, that 64% of those who had high office and ambulatory pressures had advanced changes in the optic fundi and on the ECG, but among those with high office pressures, but low ambulatory pressures only 19% had such changes. Parati et al. (83), also using the Oxford technique, found less severe grades of abnormalities in the ECG, optic fundi, and renal function in those patients whose ambulatory pressures were lower than their office pressures than in those with higher ambulatory, but equivalent office, pressures. Patients with low ambulatory pressures had 30 to 50% less target organ damage than did those with higher ambulatory pressures, except for the patients with the highest office pressures in whom the level of the ambulatory pressure did not discriminate between levels of severity. Contrary to the experience of others, Parati and coworkers (83) found a positive correlation between the variability of the ambulatory pressure and the degree of abnormality.

Several investigators have related left ventricular mass, as determined by echocardiography, to blood pressure levels (126). Rowlands et al. (102) reported that left ventricular mass index correlated better with 24-hr ambulatory mean pressure than with office pressure, $r = .60$ for ambulatory systolic and $r = .43$ for ambulatory diastolic, whereas $r = .51$ for office systolic and $r = .30$ for office diastolic. Devereux and his coworkers (19) found the highest correlation of left ventricular mass index with the pressures obtained at work, $r = .50$ for systolic and $r = .39$ for diastolic at work but the correlation with office and with home pressures was only $r = .24$ and .20 for systolic and diastolic pressures in the office and $r = .32$ and .21 for the corresponding pressures at home. Alicandri and coworkers (3) reported that average 24-hr intra-arterial pressures were significantly higher in hypertensive patients with left ventricular hypertrophy than in those without. Other investigators have reported that both the 24-hr and the exercise blood pressure correlate better with the presence of left ventricular hypertrophy than do the office pressures (20,38,120).

In subsequent studies we observed that among patients with equivalent office blood pressures, those who had lower ambulatory pressures not only had less evidence of target organ damage but were less likely to have suffered a clinical cardiovascular event such as a myocardial infarct, stroke, acceleration of hypertension, or renal impairment (85,87,90,113). For instance, among patients whose office diastolic pressure ranged between 90 and 99 mmHg, nearly 80% of those whose ambulatory mean was below 80 mmHg were in severity class 0 (no evidence of target organ involvement), 23% of those with ambulatory pressures between 80 and 89 mmHg were class 0, but only 10% of those with ambulatory pressures of 90 mmHg or above were free of target organ abnormalities (88). Similarly, among patients whose office diastolic pressure was between 110 and 119 mmHg, 29% of those with ambulatory pressures below 100 mmHg were class 0, but all of the patients with ambulatory pressures of 110 mmHg or higher were in severity class II or III (90).

RELATIONSHIP OF BLOOD PRESSURE LEVEL TO EMOTIONS AND MOODS

Repetitive measurements throughout the day also facilitate the correlation of specific activities, moods, and emotions with variations in the blood pressure (26,35,44,55). Because of our previous interest in the response to stress of college women with borderline hypertension, we analyzed the relationship of changes in blood pressure with changes in mood, as reported in the log of activities kept by the patient, and a postmonitoring interview (85). We observed a close correlation between those moods that we combined under the term *negative affect* and rises in blood pressure (44,115). Pressures were higher when the patients were in a group or talking, than when they were alone and silent (85). Similar observations have been reported by James and coworkers (55). However, the correlation of activities, moods, and emotions with concurrent blood pressure levels has been addressed only in a preliminary form; these stimuli are difficult to quantitate, and people vary widely in their responses to the same subjective stimuli.

PROGNOSTIC VALUE OF AMBULATORY BLOOD PRESSURES

We were particularly interested in the large and unexpected disparity between office and ambulatory pressures observed in some individuals. Although in the group as a whole there was a significant correlation between the average office and ambulatory pressures (r = .65), in the majority the ambulatory pressures were lower than the office pressures, and in some individuals the disparity was considerable. The disparity between office and ambulatory pressure increased with increasing office blood pressure and with increasing age, especially in women (113). We had previously observed in a study on the natural history of essential hypertension that, although the higher the pressure on the initial visit the greater the 5-year mortality, there was a significant number of patients, mostly white women, who survived without complications for more than 5 years, despite the initially high pressures (112). We speculated whether those patients with high initial pressures who unexpectedly survived actually had had lower pressures during the remainder of the day. A number of these long survivors subsequently had ambulatory blood pressure monitoring, and indeed, many of them had much lower ambulatory than office pressures. However, these retrospective results can only be considered anecdotal.

To explore this theory further, a prospective study was initiated to determine if ambulatory pressures correlated better with long-term prognosis than did office pressures; in other words, if among patients with equivalent office pressures and other risk factors, those with the lower ambulatory pressures would survive longer and have fewer cardiovascular complications than individuals with higher ambulatory pressures.

This study included all patients from the University of California at San Francisco Ambulatory Blood Pressure Laboratory on whom adequate initial clinical data were available, including an ambulatory recording and multiple concurrent office blood pressure readings (86). Patients wore the ambulatory blood pressure recorder on 1 to 3 consecutive weekdays that were intended to be representative of their usual activities. However, we did not try to standardize the patients' activities during the day. Patients included housewives who "worked" at home, professionals who came home at the end of the day, students and nurses who attended classes, retirees, and laborers. Some exercised vigorously, others took a day off from work and watched television.

After the ambulatory recording was completed, baseline clinical data had been obtained, and secondary hypertension had been excluded, the patients were entered into a treatment program and were managed on the basis of their office pressures, using the best available drug therapy or life-style modification, as indicated. Therapy was selected to reduce office pressures below 140/90 mmHg if possible, with a minimum of side effects. Most patients were followed by the authors, at the Hypertension Clinic of the University of California at San Francisco, others were followed by their personal physicians in the greater San Francisco Bay area to whom the ambulatory blood pressure data were made available. Some patients who had low or "normal" ambulatory pressures, despite higher office pressures, were initially managed with life-style changes rather than drug therapy. Likewise in some patients who were studied while receiving therapy, physicians were satisfied with current drug regimens when ambulatory pressures indicated good control even when the office pressures remained higher. On the other hand, patients who had high office and ambulatory pressures were treated more aggressively.

Once patients were enrolled in the study and treatment program, observations on their clinical course were made and recorded periodically, at least annually. Every effort was made to determine if patients had developed a clinical cardiovascular event such as a hemorrhagic or thrombotic stroke, transient cerebral ischemic attack, manifestations of ischemic heart disease, peripheral vascular disease, renal failure, acceleration of hypertension, etc. Wayward patients who failed to return to the clinic were contacted and urged to return for follow-up care. Regular progress reports were solicited from the patients' private physicians. When patients were known to have died or been hospitalized, hospital records and death certificates were requested, to determine the premorbid events, nature of clinical complication, and date and cause of death.

Of the 1,076 patients on whom adequate data were available, 762 had their first study before the initiation of therapy and 314 were receiving antihypertensive therapy at the time of the first study. The sexes were equally represented, two-thirds were younger than 50 years at entry, with the mean age for the group being 44.5 ± 14.1 years, and two-thirds were white, with the remainder black, Latino, or Asian. Most of the patients had mild hypertension with three-fourths having normal or only minimal changes in the optic fundi, two-thirds had a normal heart size on roentgenogram of the chest, and only one-fifth had evidence of LVH by ECG. The average office pressure for the group was 161.2 ± 22.6 mmHg systolic and 100.7 ± 12.1 mmHg diastolic. The average interval from entry until the first clinical cardiovascular event was 4.9 ± 3.5 years. For patients who remained event-free, the average duration of follow-up was 5.1 ± 3.5 years (86).

The clinical outcome was analyzed in terms of the development of new clinical events such as ischemic cardiac, cerebral, or peripheral vascular disease, cerebral hemorrhage, congestive failure, acceleration of hypertension, aortic dissection, renal failure, retinal arterial or venous occlusion, etc. Nonfatal events occurred in 153 patients and 75 died during the total period of follow-up of up to 10 years. The majority of these were manifestations of ischemic heart disease and one-third were due to cerebral events. Patients were subdivided into those who had not suffered a clinical cardiovascular event before entry into the study (851) and those who had (225). Of the former, 12.5% developed a cardiovascular complication, 2.8% fatal and 9.6% nonfatal during the total period of follow-up. Of the patients with prior cardiovascular complications, 54.2% developed an event, 22.7% fatal, and 31.6% nonfatal. Patients who had not had a prior event and who did not develop an event during the 10-year period of follow-up, were younger, had lower blood pressures, both ambulatory and in the office, both systolic and diastolic, and had a shorter duration of hypertension on average. The incidence of new events increased in a stepwise manner among patients with each higher level of entry blood pressure, each added decade, each successive severity grade of funduscopic findings, and degree of LVH as determined from the ECG or roentgenogram. The prognostic indicators previously described by our group and by others were thus again validated (58,103,112), although this group of patients had relatively mild hypertension and most received drug therapy, and the total number of deaths was small.

The next step was to determine if ambulatory blood pressure measurements contributed additional predictive information to that provided by the previously recognized risk factors, and if the disparity between office and ambulatory pressures could explain the unexpected survival of some patients with initially high office pressures. Although there was a reasonably linear correlation between office and ambulatory pressures for the group of patients as a whole, $r = .69$ for systolic and $r = .64$ for diastolic, ambulatory pressures were lower than office pressures in 78% of patients and ambulatory pressures could not be predicted from the office pressures for the individual patient.

To relate ambulatory pressures to office pressures, and to facilitate making comparisons between individual patients with equivalent office pressures but different ambulatory pressures, we calculated an "expected" ambulatory pressure for each patient. This was calculated from that patient's office pressure and the regression equation derived from regressing ambulatory pressure on office pressure for the entire group of patients. Patients were then classified into three groups on the basis of the difference between their observed and their calculated ambulatory pressures: those whose observed ambulatory pressures were 10 or more mmHg systolic or 6 or more mmHg diastolic above the calculated ambulatory pressure (high group), or below the calculated ambulatory level (low group), or within 9/5 mmHg of the calculated pressure (intermediate group). We used the life-table method of recording outcome and graphed the cumulative incidence of new clinical cardiovascular events over 10 years for each of these groups of patients.

Patients with "high" ambulatory pressures had a greater cumulative incidence of new fatal and nonfatal cardiovascular events, and developed them sooner than did the patients in the "low" ambulatory pressure group (86–88). Table 1 gives the *p* values for the statistical differences (using the log rank method of analysis) between the life events curves for the high and low ambulatory blood pressure groups subdivided further by office pressure, sex, age, severity of disease, and presence or absence of prior cardiovascular events. The differences in outcome between the high and low ambulatory groups were significant at the $p<.05$ level in all subgroups, for both systolic and diastolic pressures, except in patients with prior events, patients over the age of 50 years at entry, patients with office diastolic pressure greater than 105 mmHg at entry, and for diastolic pressure in women (86).

TABLE 1. *Statistical differences in 10-year cumulative incidence of cardiovascular events in patient with higher versus lower observed ambulatory blood pressures*[a]

Subgroup	Systolic	Diastolic
All patients (total events)	0.00005	0.005
All patients (deaths)	0.003	0.002
No prior CVE[b]	0.0006	0.007
With prior CVE	0.130	0.355
OBP[c] $<$ 160/105 mmHg	0.007	0.012
OBP $>$ 160/105 mmHg	0.002	0.081
Age $\leq$ 50 years	0.003	0.01
Age $\geq$ 50 years	0.051	0.108
Severity class 0–I[d]	0.002	0.017
Severity class II or more	0.017	0.430
Women	0.001	0.177
Men	0.014	0.006

[a]In relation to the calcualted ambulatory pressure.
[b]CVE, cardiovascular events.
[c]OBP, office blood pressure.
[d]Class, severity of hypertension (see ref. 86).

Figures 1, 2, and 3 are examples of these life events curves in patients whose observed ambulatory systolic pressure was 10 mmHg or whose observed ambulatory diastolic pressure was 6 mmHg above or below the level calculated from the regression equation (RE). In these three figures the patients are further subdivided by sex (Fig. 1), age (Fig. 2), and severity class (Fig. 3). In this analysis ambulatory blood pressures provided additional prognostic information to that obtained from the office pressure, by discriminating between higher and lower risk groups, especially in younger patients, in patients with mild disease, and in patients without prior clinical events, the very group of patients in whom the decision to initiate antihypertensive therapy is most controversial (86).

We performed a subsequent analysis on the subgroup of 761 patients whose initial ambulatory recording was performed before antihypertensive therapy was initiated (89). Because of the powerful independent effect on outcome of the presence of prior cardiovascular events, we subdivided this sample into the 695 who had not suffered a clinical cardiovascular event and the 102 who had. In this analysis we used the Cox proportional hazards model of analysis in order to determine the independent incremental effect of each of the following factors that could influence outcome: sex, age, ECG evidence of LVH, hypertensive retinopathy, office and ambulatory pressures, the "residual pressure" (the difference between the observed and the calculated ambulatory pressure), and subsequent drug therapy (89). In the subgroup without prior events the following characteristics were independently predictive of a low incidence of events: female sex, young age, low office systolic pressure, and residual ambulatory systolic pressure, as well as absence of advanced ECG-LVH. In those with prior events, only female sex, young age, residual ambulatory systolic pressure, and use of anti-

FIG. 1. Estimated cumulative 10-year incidence of a first clinical cardiovascular (CV) event, fatal or nonfatal, among hypertensive women and men subdivided according to the difference between their observed and their predicted ambulatory blood pressure, above or below the regression equation (RE) or predicted ambulatory pressure.

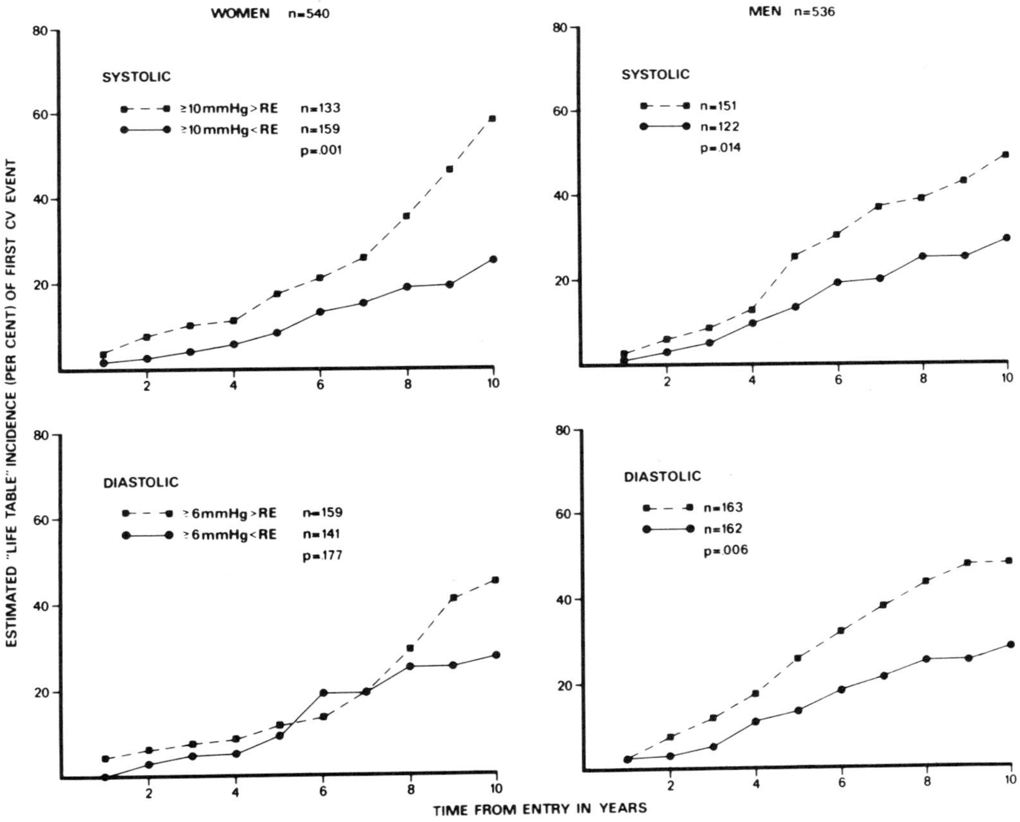
WOMEN n=540
MEN n=536
SYSTOLIC
≥10 mmHg > RE n=133
≥10 mmHg < RE n=159
p=.001
n=151
n=122
p=.014
DIASTOLIC
≥6 mmHg > RE n=159
≥6 mmHg < RE n=141
p=.177
n=163
n=162
p=.006
ESTIMATED "LIFE TABLE" INCIDENCE (PER CENT) OF FIRST CV EVENT
TIME FROM ENTRY IN YEARS

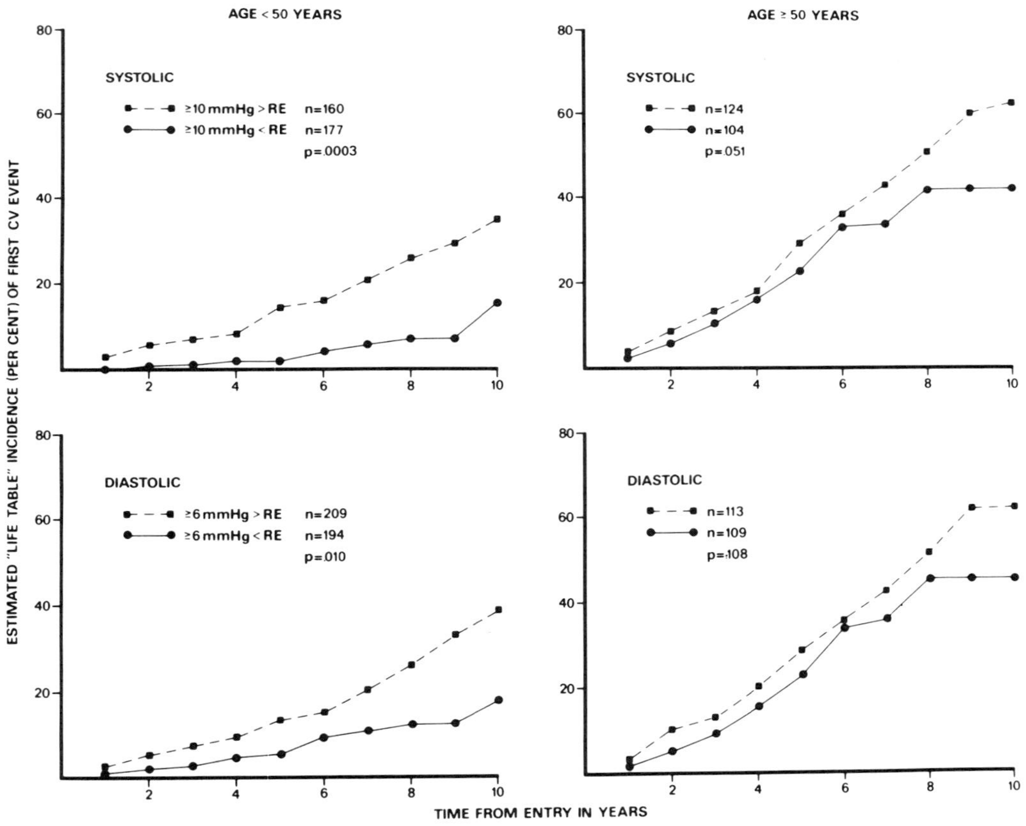

AGE < 50 YEARS
AGE ≥ 50 YEARS
SYSTOLIC
≥10 mmHg > RE n=160
≥10 mmHg < RE n=177
p=.0003
n=124
n=104
p=.051
DIASTOLIC
≥6 mmHg > RE n=209
≥6 mmHg < RE n=194
p=.010
n=113
n=109
p=.108
ESTIMATED "LIFE TABLE" INCIDENCE (PER CENT) OF FIRST CV EVENT
TIME FROM ENTRY IN YEARS
0
20
40
60
80
2
4
6
8
10

hypertensive therapy were independently predictive of a longer event-free survival period. This later study thus confirmed the independent predictive role of ambulatory pressures, with all other risk factors controlled, even in patients with prior cardiovascular complications (89). The risk of developing cardiovascular events increased with each increment of residual systolic ambulatory pressure both in those with and without prior clinical events, when all other risk factors were held constant (89).

An analysis of 459 patients who were studied while on drug treatment yielded similar results, with a significant difference in outcome between those individuals who had high ambulatory pressures compared to those with low ambulatory pressures, even though they had equivalent office pressures (88). In this group the independent predictive value of high office pressures, evidence of left ventricular hypertrophy on the electrocardiogram, advanced changes in the optic fundi (Keith Wagener classification II or more), and presence of prior cardiovascular events was again confirmed (88).

To assess whether it was the subsequent blood pressure control, rather than the initial ambulatory blood pressure, that determined if patients would develop clinical events, we reviewed the follow-up blood pressure data on 106 patients, who were under the age of 60 when first studied and whose ambulatory blood pressures were less than 140/90 mmHg, although they had been referred to as "hypertensives" (87). Nearly 80% of these individuals were subsequently given antihypertensive therapy despite their initial low ambulatory readings. Their average office blood pressure declined from 149/96 to 140/89 mmHg, and in the 46 who had follow-up ambulatory readings, the average ambulatory pressures was 126/80 mmHg initially and 127/83 mmHg subsequently. Of the 106 patients only four developed a cardiovascular complication during the follow-up period. The initial and follow-up office readings of these four were 146/102 and 145/99 mmHg, respectively, and the average ambula-

FIG. 2. Estimated cumulative 10-year incidence of a first clinical cardiovascular (CV) event, fatal, or nonfatal, among hypertensive patients grouped by age and subdivided according to the difference between their observed and their predicted ambulatory blood pressure, above or below the regression equation (RE).

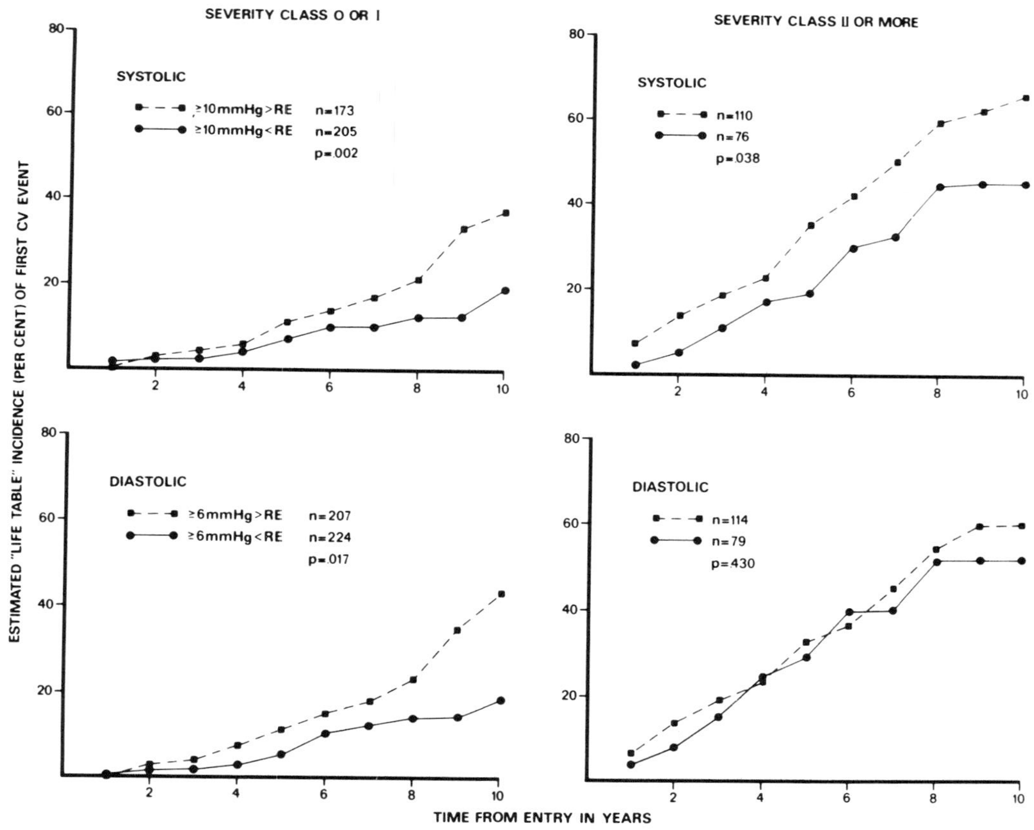
SEVERITY CLASS O OR I
SYSTOLIC
≥10mmHg>RE n=173
≥10mmHg<RE n=205
p=.002
DIASTOLIC
≥6mmHg>RE n=207
≥6mmHg<RE n=224
p=.017
SEVERITY CLASS II OR MORE
SYSTOLIC
n=110
n=76
p=.038
DIASTOLIC
n=114
n=79
p=430
ESTIMATED "LIFE TABLE" INCIDENCE (PER CENT) OF FIRST CV EVENT
TIME FROM ENTRY IN YEARS
80
60
40
20
2
4
6
8
10

tory pressure was 131/86 initially and 125/88 on follow-up. These data suggest that an initial low ambulatory reading is predictive of a relatively benign subsequent course, and ease of blood pressure control. However, the additive effect of other risk factors for atherosclerosis must be kept in mind (87).

Similar results have been reported by Mann and coworkers (73) who evaluated 137 patients with both ambulatory and office pressures and followed them for 1 to 4 years, average 23.2 months, using conventional antihypertensive therapy. Clinical cardiovascular events occurred in 14 patients. The authors used simple and multiple logistic regression analyses to test various indices for their power to distinguish the groups of patients with abnormal preexisting features and those who developed events. All indices of mean blood pressure discriminated between groups. The 24-hr mean ambulatory pressure had greater predictive power than the office pressure in eight out of ten comparisons. Nighttime and morning pressures were more predictive of outcome than were pressures averaged for the afternoon or evening. Clinic systolic and diastolic pressures were equally predictive of severity and of outcome, whereas ambulatory systolic pressures were more predictive than were ambulatory diastolic pressures. Blood pressure variability had no independent predictive power (73).

In summary, the lessons to be learned from ambulatory blood pressure monitoring can be stated as follows: Hypertension leads progressively to morbidity and death from cardiovascular disease. The higher the blood pressure, the greater is the likelihood and degree of abnormality in the cardiovascular target organs. The more advanced the evidence of target organ damage, the greater is the morbidity and mortality. Ambulatory blood pressures correlate better with the degree of target organ damage than do office blood pressures, in the individual patient. Therefore, ambulatory pres-

FIG. 3. Estimated cumulative 10-year incidence of a first clinical cardiovascular (CV) event, fatal or nonfatal, among hypertensive patients grouped by severity class and subdivided according to the difference between their observed and their predicted ambulatory blood pressure, above or below the regression equation (RE).

sures should correlate better with outcome than office pressures. We have shown that ambulatory pressures are independent predictors of risk for the development of clinical events. Therefore, in patients with equivalent office pressures, those with the higher ambulatory pressures are more likely to develop cardiovascular complications than are those with lower ambulatory pressures.

However, the development of cardiovascular disease is accelerated by multiple risk factors in addition to an elevated blood pressure, such as advancing age, a positive family history of premature cardiovascular disease, cigarette smoking, hyperlipidemia, diabetes mellitus, inadequacy of antihypertensive therapy, and others (103). All of these risk factors must be taken into consideration in decisions regarding the individual patient. Thus, since hypertension is a quantitative disease, not an all-or-none phenomenon, as was so aptly pointed out by Sir George Pickering, and since there is no clear dividing line between risk and no risk, each patient must be treated individually and all of the available information considered in the decisions regarding management. Ambulatory blood pressures contribute to that risk assessment by amplifying the blood pressure information, but these measurements also must be considered in the context of the total picture.

REFERENCES

1. Addis T. Blood pressure and pulse rate levels: I. The levels under basal and daytime conditions. *Arch Intern Med* 1922;29:539–553.
2. Alam GM, Smirk FH. Casual and basal blood pressures: II. In essential hypertension. *Br Heart J* 1943;5:156–161.
3. Alicandri C, Fariello R, Boni E, Muiesan ML, Zanielli A, Agabiti-Rosei E, Muiesan G. Left ventricular hypertrophy and ambulatory monitoring of blood pressure. *J Clin Hypertens* 1987;3:197–202.
4. Armitage P, Fox W, Rose GA, Tinker CM. The variability of measurements of casual blood pressure: II. Survey experience. *Clin Sci* 1966;30:337–344.
5. Armitage P, Rose GA. The variability of measurements of casual blood pressure. I. A laboratory study. *Clin Sci* 1966;30:325–335.
6. Australian National Blood Pressure Study Management Committee. The Australian therapeutic trial in mild hypertension. *Lancet* 1980;1:1261–1267.
7. Ayman D, Goldshine AD. Blood pressure determinations by patients with essential hypertension: I. The difference between clinic and home readings before treatment. *Am J Med Sci* 1940;200:465–474.

8. Bevan AT, Honour AJ, Stott FD. Direct arterial pressure recording in unrestricted man. *Clin Sci* 1969;36:329–344.
9. Breslin DJ, Gifford RW Jr, Fairbairn JF II, Kairns TP. Prognostic importance of ophthalmoscopic findings in essential hypertension. *JAMA* 1966; 195:335–338.
10. Brunner HR, Waeber B, Nussberger J. Blood pressure recording in the ambulatory patient and evaluation of cardiovascular risk. *Clin Sci* 1985;68:485–488.
11. Burstyn P, Donovan B, Charlton I. Blood pressure variability: the effects of repeated measurements. *Postgrad Med J* 1981;57:488–491.
12. Carey RM, Reid RA, Ayers CR, Lynch SS, McLain WL, Vaughan ED Jr. The Charlottesville blood-pressure survey: Value of repeated blood-pressure measurements. *JAMA* 1976;236:847–851.
13. Casale, PN, Devereux RB, Milner M, Zullo G, Harshfield GA, Pickering TG, Laragh JH. Value of echocardiographic measurement of left ventricular mass in predicting cardiovascular morbid events in hypertensive men. *Ann Intern Med* 1986;105:173–178.
14. Castelli WP. Epidemiology of coronary heart disease: the Framingham Study. *Am J Med* 1984;76(suppl 2A):4–12.
15. Cheung D, Weber MA. Ambulatory blood pressure measurements: practical considerations, methodology, feasibility, and implications in the management of hypertension. *Cardiovasc Clin* 1988;18:125–138.
16. Clement DL, Mussche MM, Vanhoutte G, Pannier R. Is blood pressure variability related to activity of the sympathetic system? *Clin Sci* 1979;57 (suppl):217s–219s.
17. Cowan RM, Sokolow M, Perloff D. Methodological consideration in determining the accuracy of an indirect blood pressure recorder. In: Stott FD, Raftery EB, Goulding, L, eds. *Proceedings of the Third International Symposium on Ambulatory Monitoring*. New York: Academic Press, 1980;241–247.
18. Cox J, O'Malley K, Atkins N, O'Brien E. A comparison of the twenty-four hour blood pressure profile in normotensive and hypertensive subjects. *J Hypertens* 1991;9(suppl 1):S3–S6.
19. Devereux RB, Pickering TG, Harshfield GA, Kleinert HD, Denby L, Clark L, Pregibon D, Jason M, Kleiner B, Borer JS, Laragh JH. Left ventricular hypertrophy in patients with hypertension: Importance of blood pressure response to regularly recurring stress. *Circulation* 1983;68:470–476.
20. Dimitriou R, De Gaudemaris R, Debru JL, Dubois F, Camaleonte A, Pedrix A, Mallion JM. Data on the echocardiogram, pressure profile during exertion, and ambulatory blood pressure measurements in borderline arterial hypertension. *Arch Mal Coeur* 1984;77:1162–1166.
21. Di Rienzo M, Grassi G, Pedotti A, Mancia G. Continuous vs intermittent blood pressure measurements in estimating 24-average blood pressure. *Hypertension* 1983;5:264–269.
22. Di Rienzo M, Parati G, Pomidossi G, Veniani M, Pedotti A, Mancia G. Blood pressure monitoring over short day and night times cannot predict 24-hour average blood pressure. *J Hypertens* 1983;3:343–349.
23. Drayer JI, Gardin JM, Brewer DD, Weber MA. Disparate relationships between blood pressure and left ventricular mass in patients with and without left ventricular hypertrophy. *Hypertension* 1987;9(2 pt.2):II61–II64.

24. Dupont AG, Vanderniepen P, Volckaert A, Finne E, Six RO. Noninvasive ambulatory monitoring of blood pressure in essential hypertension. Effect of age on variability and disparity. *J Clin Hypertens* 1986;2:278–284.
25. Dyken ML, Wolf PA, Barnett HJM, Bergan JJ, Hass WK, Kannel WB, Kuller L, Kurtzke JF, Sundt TM. Risk factors in stroke: a statement for physicians by the Subcommittee on Risk Factors and Stroke of the Stroke Council. *Stroke* 1984;15:1105–1111.
26. Eliasson K, Hjemdahl P, Kahan T. Circulatory and sympathoadrenal responses to stress in borderline and established hypertension. *J Hypertens* 1983;1:131–139.
27. Floras JS, Hassan MO, Jones JV, Osikowska BA, Sever PS, Sleight P. Factors influencing blood pressure and heart rate variability in hypertensive humans. *Hypertension* 1988;11:273–281.
28. Floras JS, Jones JV, Hassan MO, Osikowska B, Sever, PS, Sleight P. Cuff and ambulatory blood pressure in subjects with essential hypertension. *Lancet* 1981;2:107–109.
29. Freis ED. The discrepancy between home and office recordings of blood pressure in patients treated with pentapyrrolidinium: importance of home recordings in adjusting dosage. *Med Ann DC* 1954;23:363–367.
30. Freis ED and the Veterans Administration Cooperative Study Group on Antihypertensive Agents. Effects of treatment on morbidity in hypertension: I. Results in patients with diastolic blood pressures averaging 115 through 129 mm Hg. *JAMA* 1967;202:1028–1034.
31. Frielingsdorf J, Stricker M, Hany St, Foerster CCh, Vetter W. 24-Stunden Blutdruckmessung bei Hypertonien verschiedener Schweregrade. *Schweiz Rundsch Med Prax* 1985;74:1260–1265.
32. Frohlich E, Tarazi R. Is arterial pressure the sole factor responsible for hypertensive cardiac hypertrophy? *Am J Cardiol* 1979;44:959–963.
33. Froom P, Bar-David M, Ribak J, Van Dyk D, Kallner B, Benbassat J. Predictive value of systolic blood pressure in young men for elevated systolic blood pressure 12 to 15 years later. *Circulation* 1983;68:467–469.
34. Garrett BN, Salcedo JR, Thompson AM. The role of ambulatory blood pressure monitoring in the evaluation of adolescent hypertension. *Clin Exp Hypertens* 1985;7:227–234.
35. Germanó G, Ferrucci A, Strano S, Molle G, Napoleoni MG, Pecchioli V, Germanó U, Pistone A. Pressor effects from daily events and laboratory complex stimuli relating personality factors. *Clin Cardiol* 1987;10:659–664.
36. Glock CY, Vought RL, Clark EG, Schweitzer MD. Studies in hypertension. II. Variability of daily blood pressure measurements in the same individuals over a three-week period. *J Chron Dis* 1956;4:469–476.
37. Gordon T, Sorlie P, Kannel WB. Problems in the assessment of blood pressure: the Framingham study. *Int J Epidemiol* 1976;5:327–334.
38. Gosse P, Campello G, Aouizerate E, Roudaut R, Dallocchio M. Left ventricular hypertrophy of the hypertensive patient: relation to exertional and ambulatory blood pressure. *Arch Mal Coeur* 1986;79:796–800.
39. Gosse P, Campello G, Roudaut R, Aouizerate E, Dallocchio M. Should nocturnal arterial pressure be monitored in treated hypertensive patients? *Arch Mal Coeur* 1987;80:1011–1014.
40. Gould BA, Hornung RS, Altman DG, Cashman PMM, Raftery E. Indirect

measurement of blood pressure during exercise testing can be misleading. *Br Heart J* 1985;53:611–615.

41. Gould BA, Hornung RS, Kieso HA, Altman DG, Cashman PM, Raftery EB. Evaluation of the Remler M2000 blood pressure recorder. Comparison with intraarterial blood pressure recordings both at hospital and at home. *Hypertension* 1984;6(2 pt. 1):209–215.
42. Gould BA, Hornung RS, Kieso H, Cashman PMM, Raftery EB. An evaluation of self-recorded blood pressure during drug trials. *Hypertension* 1986;8: 267–271.
43. Hany St, Baumgart P, Baettig B, Valger P, Vetter W, Vetter H. Diagnostische Aspekte der 24-Stunden-Blutdruckmessung. *Schweiz Rundsch Med Prax* 1987;76:480–584.
44. Harris RE, Sokolow M, Carpenter LG Jr, Freedman M, Hunt SP. Response to psychologic stress in persons who are potentially hypertensive. *Circulation* 1953;7:874–879.
45. Health and Public Policy Committee, American College of Physicians. Automated ambulatory blood pressure monitoring. *Ann Intern Med* 1986;104: 275–278.
46. Hines EA. Range of normal blood pressure and subsequent development of hypertension; follow-up study of 1,522 patients. *JAMA* 1940;115:271–274.
47. Hinman AT, Engel BT, Bickford AF. Portable blood pressure recorder: accuracy and preliminary use in evaluating intradaily variations in pressure. *Am Heart J* 1962;63:663–668.
48. Hoefling B. Ambulante programmierte Blutduckmessung ueber 24 Stunden. *Fortschr Med* 1987;105:473–476.
49. Horan MJ, Padgett NE, Kennedy HL. Ambulatory blood pressure monitoring: recent advances and clinical applications. *Am Heart J* 1981;101:843–848.
50. Hossman V, Fitzgerald GA, Dollery CT. Influence of hospitalization and placebo therapy on blood pressure and sympathetic function in essential hypertension. *Hypertension* 1981;3:113–118.
51. Hypertension Detection and Follow-up Program. Five-year findings of the Hypertension Detection and Follow-up Program: I. Reduction in mortality of persons with high blood pressure, including mild hypertension. *JAMA* 1979;242:2562–2571.
52. Ibrahim MM, Tarazi RC, Dustan HP, Gifford RW. Electrocardiogram in evaluation of resistance to antihypertensive therapy. *Arch Intern Med* 1977; 137:1125–1129.
53. Irving JB, Kerr F, Ewing DJ, Kirby BJ. Value of prolonged recording of blood pressure in assessment of hypertension. *B Heart J* 1974;36:859–866.
54. Jacot des Combes B, Porchet M, Waeber B, Brunner HR. Ambulatory blood pressure recordings. Reproducibility and unpredictability. *Hypertension* 1984;6:110–114.
55. James GD, Yee LS, Harshfield GA, Blank SG, Pickering TG. The influence of happiness, anger, and anxiety on the blood pressure of borderline hypertensives. *Psychosom Med* 1986;48:502–508.
56. Julius S, Ellis CN, Pascual AV, Matice M, Hansson L, Hunyor SN, Sandler LN. Home blood pressure determination. Value in borderline ("labile") hypertension. *JAMA* 1974;229:663–666.

57. Kain HR, Hinman AT, Sokolow M. Arterial blood pressure measurements with a portable blood pressure recorder in hypertensive patients: I. Variability and correlation with "casual" pressures. *Circulation* 1964;30:882–892.
58. Kannel WB. Role of blood pressure in cardiovascular morbidity and mortality. *Prog Cardiovasc Dis* 1974;17:5–24.
59. Kannel WB. Prevalence and natural history of electrocardiographic left ventricular hypertrophy. *Am J Med* 1983;75(suppl 3A):3A4–3A11.
60. Kannel WB, Sorlie P, Gordon T. Labile hypertension: a faulty concept? The Framingham study. *Circulation* 1980;61:1183–1187.
61. Kaplan NM. Misdiagnosis of systemic hypertension and recommendations for improvement. *Am J Cardiol* 1987;60:1383–1386.
62. Kennedy HL, Horan MJ, Sprague MK, Padgett NE, Shriver KK. Ambulatory blood pressure in healthy normotensive males. *Am Heart J* 1983;106: 717–722.
63. Kobrin I, Oigman W, Kumar A, Ventura HO, Messerli FH, Frohlich ED, Dunn FG. Diurnal variation of blood pressure in elderly patients with essential hypertension. *J Am Geriatr Soc* 1984;32:896–899.
64. Kooperstein SI, Schifrin A, Leahy TJ. Level of initial blood pressure and subsequent development of essential hypertension. A ten and fifteen year follow-up study. *Am J Cardiol* 1962;10:416–423.
65. Levy RL, Hillman CC, Stroud WD, White PD. Transient hypertension: its significance in terms of later development of sustained hypertension and cardiovascular-renal diseases. *JAMA* 1944;120:829–833.
66. Linsell CR, Lightman SL, Mullen PE, Brown MJ, Causon RC. Circadian rhythms of epinephrine and norepinephrine in man. *J Clin Endocrinol Metab* 1985;60:1210–1215.
67. Littler WA, Honour AJ, Pugsley DJ, Sleight P. Continuous recording of direct arterial pressure in unrestricted patients: its role in the diagnosis and management of high blood pressure. *Circulation* 1975;51:1101–1106.
68. Littler WA, Honour AJ, Sleight P, Stott FD. Continuous recording of direct arterial pressure and electrocardiogram in unrestricted man. *Br Med J* 1972;3:76–78.
69. Mallion JM, Debru JL, De Gaudemaris R, Dimitriou R, Perdrix A, Cau G. Mesure ambulatoire de la pression artérielle: intérêt diagnostique, prognostique et thérapeutique. *Presse Med* 1985;14:151–155.
70. Mancia G, Ferrari A, Gregorini L, Parati G, Pomidossi G, Bertinieri G, Grassi G, Di Rienzo M, Pedotti A, Zanchetti A. Blood pressure and heart rate variabilities in normotensive and hypertensive human beings. *Circ Res* 1983;53:96–104.
71. Mancia G, Parati G, Pomidossi G, Grassi G, Casadei R, Zanchetti A. Alerting reaction and rise in blood pressure during measurement by physician and nurse. *Hypertension* 1987;9:209–215.
72. Mann S, Millar Craig MW, Melville DI, Balasubramanian V, Raftery EB. Physical activity and the circadian rhythm of blood pressure. *Clin Sci* 1979;57:291s–294s.
73. Mann S, Millar Craig MW, Raftery EB. Superiority of 24-hour measurement of blood pressure over clinic values in determining prognosis in hypertension. *Clin Exp Hypertens* 1985;A7(2&3):279–281.
74. Medical Research Council Working Party on Mild to Moderate Hyperten-

sion. Randomised controlled trial for mild hypertension: design and pilot trial. *Br Med J* 1977;i:1437–1440.

75. Messerli FH, Glade LB, Ventura HO, Dreslinski GR, Suarez DH, MacPhee AA, Aristimuno GG, Cole FE, Frohlich ED. Diurnal variations of cardiac rhythm, arterial pressure, and urinary catecholamines in borderline and established hypertension. *Am Heart J* 1982;104:109–114.
76. Meyer-Sabellek W, Schulte K-L, Distler A, Gotzen R. Technische Aspekte der ambulanten automatischen, nichtinvasiven 24-Stunden Blutdruckmessung. *Schweiz Rundsch Med Prax* 1987;76:443–449.
77. Montsos SE, Sapira JD, Scheib ET, Shapiro AP. An analysis of the placebo effect in hospitalized hypertensive patients. *Clin Pharmacol Ther* 1967;8: 676–683.
78. Moore-Ede MC, Czeisler CA, Richardson GS. Circadian timekeeping in health and disease: Part 1. Basic properties of circadian pacemakers. *N Engl J Med* 1983;309:469–476. Part 2. Clinical implications of circadian rhythmicity. 1983;309:530–536.
79. Nishimura H, Nishioka A, Kubo S, Suwa M, Kino M, Kawamura K. Multifactorial evaluation of blood pressure fall upon hospitalization in essential hypertensive patients. *Clin Sci* 1987;73:135–141.
80. O'Brien E, Mee F, Atkins N, O'Malley K. Inaccuracy of seven popular sphygmomanometers for home measurement of blood pressure. *J Hypertens* 1990;8:621–634.
81. O'Brien E, O'Malley K. Evaluation of blood pressure measuring devices with special reference to ambulatory systems. *J Hypertens* 1990;8(suppl 7):S133–S139.
82. Padfield PL, Lindsay BA, McLaren JA, Pirie A, Rademaker M. Changing relation between home and clinic blood-pressure measurements: Do home measurements predict clinic hypertension? *Lancet* 1987;2:322–324.
83. Parati G, Pomidossi G, Albini F, Malaspina D, Mancia G. Relationship of 24-hour blood pressure mean and variability to severity of target-organ damage in hypertension. *J Hypertens* 1987;5:93–98.
84. Parati G, Pomidossi G, Casadei R, Mancia G. Lack of alerting reactions to intermittent cuff inflations during noninvasive blood pressure monitoring. *Hypertension* 1985;7:597–601.
85. Perloff D, Sokolow M, Cowan R. Clinical relevance of ambulatory blood pressure measurements. In: Kimmich HP, ed. *Biotelemetry and patient monitoring*. Basel: S. Karger, 1981;8:67–80.
86. Perloff D, Sokolow M, Cowan R. The prognostic value of ambulatory blood pressures. *JAMA* 1983;249:2792–2798.
87. Perloff D, Sokolow M, Cowan R. Ambulatory blood pressure: the San Francisco experience. *J Hypertens* 1990;8(suppl 6):S105–S111.
88. Perloff D, Sokolow M, Cowan R. The prognostic value of ambulatory blood pressure monitoring in treated hypertensive patients. *J Hypertens* 1991;9 (suppl 1):S33–S40.
89. Perloff D, Sokolow M, Cowan R, Juster R. Prognostic value of ambulatory blood pressures; further analyses. *J Hypertens* 1989;7(suppl 3):S3–S10.
90. Perloff, D, Sokolow M, Werdegar D, Cowan RM. The value of portable blood pressure recording in guiding the treatment of hypertension. In: Dem-

ling L, Bachman K, eds. *Biotelemetrie symposium*. Stutgart: Georg Thieme Verlag, 1970;181–192.

91. Pickering G. *High blood pressure*, 2nd ed. New York: Grune and Stratton, 1968;37.
92. Pickering G. Normotension and hypertension: the mysterious viability of the false. *Am J Med* 1978;65:561–563.
93. Pickering GW, Cranston WI, Pears MA. *The treatment of hypertension*. Springfield, IL: Charles C. Thomas, 1961.
94. Pickering TG, James GD. Some implications of the differences between home, clinic and ambulatory blood pressure in normotensive and hypertensive patients. *J Hypertens* 1989;7(suppl 3):S65–S72.
95. Pickering TG, James GD, Boddie C, Harshfield GA, Blank S, Laragh JH. How common is white-coat hypertension? *JAMA* 1988;259:225–228.
96. Porchet M, Bussien JP, Waeber B, Nussberger J, Brunner HR. Unpredictability of blood pressures recorded outside the clinic in the treated hypertensive patient. *J Cardiovasc Pharmacol* 1986;8:332–335.
97. Rautaharju PM, LaCroix AZ, Savage DD, Haynes SG, Madans JH, Wolf HK, Hadden W, Keller J, Coroni-Huntley J. Electrocardiographic estimate of left ventricular mass versus radiographic cardiac size and the risk of cardiovascular disease mortality in the epidemiologic follow-up study of the First National Health and Nutrition Examination Survey. *Am J Cardiol* 1988; 62:59–66.
98. Richards AM, Nicholls MG, Espiner EA, Ikram H, Cullens M, Hinton D. Diurnal patterns of blood pressure, heart rate and vasoactive hormones in normal man. *Clin Exp Hypertens* 1986;A8:153–166.
99. Richardson DW, Honour AJ, Fenton GW, Stott FH, Pickering GW. Variation in arterial pressure throughout the day and night. *Clin Sci* 1964;26:445–460.
100. Rion F, Waeber B, Graf HJ, Jaussi A, Porchet M, Brunner HR. Blood pressure response to antihypertensive therapy: ambulatory versus office blood pressure readings. *J Hypertens* 1985;3:139–143.
101. Roberts WC. The hypertensive diseases: evidence that systemic hypertension is a greater risk factor to the development of other cardiovascular diseases than previously suspected. *Am J Med* 1975;59:523–532.
102. Rowlands DB, Ireland MA, Glover DR, McLeay RAB, Stallard TJ, Littler WA. The relationship between ambulatory blood pressure and echocardiographically assessed left ventricular hypertrophy. *Clin Sci* 1981;61:101s–103s.
103. Samuelsson O, Wilhelmsen L, Pennert K, Berglund G. Prognostic factors in treated hypertension. *J Hypertens* 1985;3(suppl 3):S497–S500.
104. Schneider RA, Kimmell GO, Van Meter AP Jr. An improved fully automatic portable blood pressure recorder. *J Appl Physiol* 1974;37:776–779.
105. Shepard DS. Reliability of blood pressure measurements: implications for designing and evaluating programs to control hypertension. *J Chron Dis* 1981; 34:191–209.
106. Sheps SG, Elveback LR, Close EL, Kleven MK, Bissen C. Evaluation of the Del Mar Avionics ambulatory blood pressure-recording device. *Mayo Clin Proc* 1981;56:740–743.
107. Smirk FH. Observations on the mortality of 270 treated and 199 untreated

retinal grade I and II hypertensive patients followed in all instances for five years. *N Z Med J* 1964;63:413–418.

108. Smirk FH, Veale AMD, Alstad KS. Basal and supplemental blood pressure in relationship to life expectancy and hypertension symptomatology. *N Z Med J* 1959;58:711–735.
109. Society of Actuaries. *Blood pressure study, 1979*. Chicago: Society of Actuaries and Association of Life Insurance Directors of America, 1980.
110. Sokolow M, Harris RE. The natural history of hypertensive disease. In: Brest AN, Moyer JH, eds. *Hypertension recent advances: The Second Hahnemann Symposium on Hypertensive Disease*. Philadelphia: Lea and Febiger, 1961; 3–23.
111. Sokolow M, Lyon TP. The ventricular complex in left ventricular hypertrophy as obtained by unipolar precordial and limb leads. *Am Heart J* 1949;37:161–186.
112. Sokolow M, Perloff D. The prognosis of essential hypertension treated conservatively. *Circulation* 1961;23:697–713.
113. Sokolow, M, Perloff D, Cowan R. Contribution of ambulatory blood pressure to the assessment of patients with mild to moderate elevation of office blood pressure. *Cardiovasc Rev Rep* 1980;1:295–303.
114. Sokolow M, Werdegar D, Kain HK, Hinman AT. Relationship between level of blood pressure measured casually and by portable recorders and severity of complications in essential hypertension. *Circulation* 1966;34:279–298.
115. Sokolow M, Werdegar D, Perloff DB, Cowan RM, Brenenstuhl H. Preliminary studies relating portably recorded blood pressures to daily life events in patients with essential hypertension. In: Koster M, Mustaph H, Visser P, eds. *Psychosomatics in essential hypertension*, no. 144. Basel/München/New York: Karger, 1970;164–189.
116. Souchek J, Stamler J, Dyer AR, Paul O, Leppert H. The value of two or three versus a single reading of blood pressure at a first visit. *J Chron Dis* 1979; 32:197–210.
117. Streitberg B. Analyse zirkadianer Blutdruckprofile—einige statistische Anmerkungen. In: Gotzen R, Meyer-Sabellek W, eds. *Indirekte 24-Stunden-Blutdruckmessung*. Darmstadt: Steinkopff Verlag, 1988;117–124.
118. Taguchi J, Freis ED. Partial reduction of blood pressure and prevention of complications in hypertension. *N Engl J Med* 1974;291:329–331.
119. Takagi N. Variability of direct arterial blood pressure in essential hypertension—relationships between the fall of blood pressure during sleep and awake resting hemodynamic parameters. *Jpn Circ J* 1986;50:587–594.
120. Vermeersch P, Duprez D, Packet L, Clement DL. Left ventricular hypertrophy in mild hypertension: value of ambulatory recordings. *J Hypertens* 1987; 5(suppl 5):S495–S496.
121. Vetter W, Schmid-Zumstein A, Baettig B, Oertel R, Hany S, Edmonds D, Baumgart P, Vetter H. 24-Stunden-Blutdruckmessung: therapeutische und prognostische Bedeutung. *Schweiz Rundsch Med Praxis* 1987;76:462–466.
122. Von Moeller J, Heyder O. Die labile Blutdrucksteigerung. *Z. Kreislauffarsch* 1959;48:413–428.
123. Waeber B, Jacot des Combes B, Porchet M. Ambulatory blood pressure recording to identify hypertensive patients who truly need therapy. *J Chron Dis* 1984;37:55–57.

124. Waeber B, Scherrer U, Petrillo A, Bidiville J, Nussberger J, Waeber G, Hofstetter JR, Brunner HR. Are some hypertensive patients overtreated? A prospective study of ambulatory blood pressure recording. *Lancet* 1987;2: 732–734.
125. Watson RDS, Stallard TJ, Flinn RM, Littler WA. Factors determining direct arterial pressure and its variability in hypertensive man. *Hypertension* 1980; 2:333–341.
126. White WB. Predicting hypertensive heart disease via non-invasive methodology: relationship between ambulatory blood pressure and cardiac indices derived by echocardiography and radionuclide ventriculography. *J Hypertens* 1990;8(suppl 6):S113–118.
127. Zachariah PK, Sheps SG, Smith RL. Clinical use of home and ambulatory blood pressure monitoring. *Mayo Clin Proc* 1989;64:1436–1446.

Ambulatory Blood Pressure Recording,
edited by H. Brunner and B. Waeber.
Raven Press, Ltd., New York © 1992.

4

How to Deal with Blood Pressure Variability

G. Parati, E. Mutti, S. Omboni, and G. Mancia

Cattedra di Semeiotica Medica and Istituto di Clinica Medica Generale e Terapia Medica, Universitá di Milano; Centro di Fisiologia Clinica e Ipertensione, Ospedale Maggiore, Milan, Italy

HISTORICAL REMARKS

The first observation that blood pressure is continuously changing over time was made by Stephen Hales in 1733, at the time of his pioneering experiments aimed at "seeing the arterial pulse." Following insertion of a glass pipe into the crural artery of a mare, Hales was so surprised by the oscillations of the blood column in the pipe as to conclude that blood pressure was likely "never to be exactly the same, any two minutes, during the whole life of an animal" (1). That blood pressure is highly variable was later confirmed by other studies, published in the 19th century by Marey, Herisson, Dudgeon et al. (2,3). These investigators drew their conclusions on blood pressure oscillations in humans from data collected by means of rudimentary noninvasive instruments devised to reproduce the arterial pulse noninvasively. Their observations were only anecdotal in nature, however, and were based on the recording of uncalibrated pulse waveform signals. The suggestion that the existence of blood pressure variations may be important also in a clinical setting was made by Scipione Riva-Rocci in 1897. In his paper, which provides the description of the sphygmomanometric technique (4), Riva-Rocci emphasized that the procedure of blood pressure measurement by the doctor was itself potentially able to induce a blood pressure rise in the patient so large as to interfere with data collection.

A more detailed analysis of blood pressure variability phenomena in humans has been made possible only in the last few decades thanks to the description of the techniques that allow blood pressure to be monitored over 24 hr in ambulatory conditions (5,6). These techniques can be subdivided into invasive or noninvasive methods. The invasive ones are most suitable for investigating blood pressure variations because they provide a continuous beat-to-beat recording of blood pressure changes throughout the monitoring period (6–8); their invasiveness, however, represents a major limitation that prevents their widespread use. This problem has stimulated the development of several noninvasive blood pressure monitoring devices that record blood pressure through intermittent inflations of an arm cuff. It has been clearly shown, however, that these systems do not provide a satisfactory tracking of blood pressure variations over a 24-hr period. Actually, besides other problems related to the accuracy of individual blood pressure readings delivered by these noninvasive monitors (9,10), the intermittency of measurements which characterizes these devices does itself represent an important limitation for studying blood pressure variability, because it is responsible for a nonnegligible loss of information on blood pressure changes of short duration (11). New perspectives for noninvasive beat-to-beat assessment of blood pressure variability have been offered by the description of a technique for continuous blood pressure recording that makes use of a small cuff wrapped around a finger of the hand (12). This technique (the Finapres technique, Ohmeda) recently has been shown to provide blood pressure values similar to those recorded intra-arterially not only at rest but also during maneuvers that quickly and markedly change blood pressure (Fig. 1) (13). A portable version of this device is under investigation. If validated, it may represent an appealing noninvasive alternative to ambulatory intra-arterial blood pressure monitoring (14).

THE ANALYSIS OF BLOOD PRESSURE VARIABILITY

If over the years several different techniques have been proposed to monitor blood pressure changes in humans, even greater is the number of methods that have been devised to quantitatively analyze

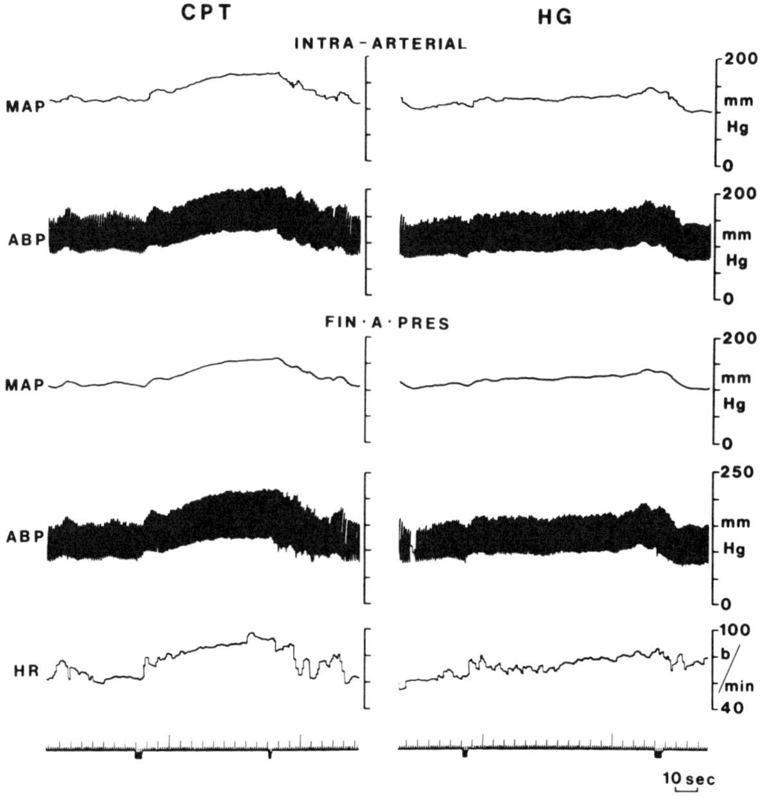

FIG. 1. Intra-arterial (*upper panels*) and finger blood pressure (Finapres, *lower panels*) tracings obtained in one subject during handgrip (HG) and cold pressor test (CPT). MAP, mean arterial pressure; ABP, pulsatile arterial blood pressure; HR, heart rate. (From ref. 13, by permission.)

blood pressure variability phenomena (6). The most widely used one is the calculation of the standard deviation (SD) of the mean blood pressure value of the recording period. This measure is simple and easy to obtain. It is also powerful, however, because, in cases of normal distribution of data, 95% of the signal is included within ± 2 SD. The major limitation of this approach is that it does not tell us anything about how single values are distributed around the mean (15). Thus, identical blood pressure means and standard deviations may correspond to thoroughly different distributions of individual values. To cope with this problem several other methods have been proposed, such as calculation of day-night difference in blood pressure, the hourly differences, the difference between peak and bottom values, etc., which may be able to provide more detailed information on the distribution of blood pressure changes over 24 hr but introduce other untoward oversimplifications in the analysis of a complex phenomenon such as blood pressure variability.

An approach that may represent a compromise between those mentioned above, and one that is currently used in our laboratory, is based on the calculation, following beat-to-beat analysis of 24-hr intra-arterial recordings, of the mean blood pressure values for each half-hour of the monitoring time with the corresponding SDs (Fig. 2). By averaging these half-hour SD values it is possible to obtain a mean "within half-hour SD," which can be taken as an index of relatively short-term blood pressure variations. On the other hand,

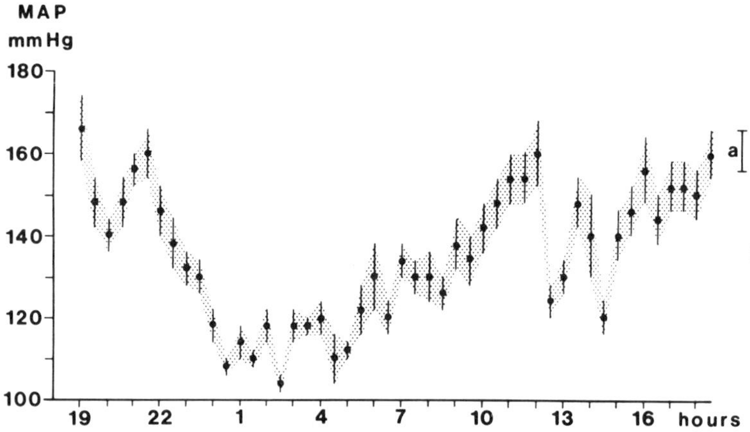

FIG. 2. Computer analysis of a 24-hr intra-arterial blood pressure recording in a hypertensive subject. *Black points* refer to average mean arterial pressure (MAP) values obtained separately for each of the 48 half-hours of the recording period, the *vertical lines* representing the corresponding standard deviations; *a* represents the average of the 48 standard deviations (one for each half-hour) and is referred to as variability within half-hours or short-term MAP variability; *b* represents the standard deviation obtained by averaging the 48 average MAP values (one for each half-hour) and is referred to as variability among half-hours or long-term MAP variability. The *horizontal line* at the bottom indicates the time during the recording. (From ref. 16, by permission.)

by averaging the half-hour mean values it is possible to compute the 24-hr mean blood pressure with its SD. This "among half-hour SD" provides information on relatively more long-term blood pressure changes (16). Besides the above-mentioned methods, other more sophisticated approaches have been proposed, either in the time or in the frequency domain, which provide more details about specific components of blood pressure variability phenomena. By means of these procedures, it is possible to separately analyze two important elements of blood pressure variability: (a) the transient irregular rises or falls in blood pressure that may be variably coupled with parallel or opposite changes in heart rate, and (b) the rhythmic oscillations in blood pressure and heart rate that are known to occur throughout any given recording period, with particular attention to those oscillations with frequencies ranging between 0.025 and 0.5 Hz (17).

GENERAL FEATURES OF BLOOD PRESSURE VARIABILITY

Studies performed by intra-arterial ambulatory blood pressure monitoring (6,16,18) have shown that over a 24-hr period blood pressure variations amount to about 10% of the mean 24-hr value. In absolute terms, systolic blood pressure variability is greater than diastolic blood pressure variability, although there are no differences when blood pressure variations are expressed as a percent of the mean value. Furthermore, long-term variability, as previously defined, is higher than short-term variability. Short-term variability is highest during the daytime and lowest during sleep, in parallel with the changes in half-hour blood pressure means (Fig. 3). This means that, in a given subject, the magnitude of within–half-hour blood pressure variations is positively related to half-hour mean blood pressure values. Similar observations have been reported also on the behavior of heart rate half-hour means and standard deviations (16). When different subjects characterized by different blood pressure levels are considered, blood pressure variability in absolute terms is higher in subjects with higher blood pressure and vice versa (6). Thus, 24-hr blood pressure SD increases progressively on going

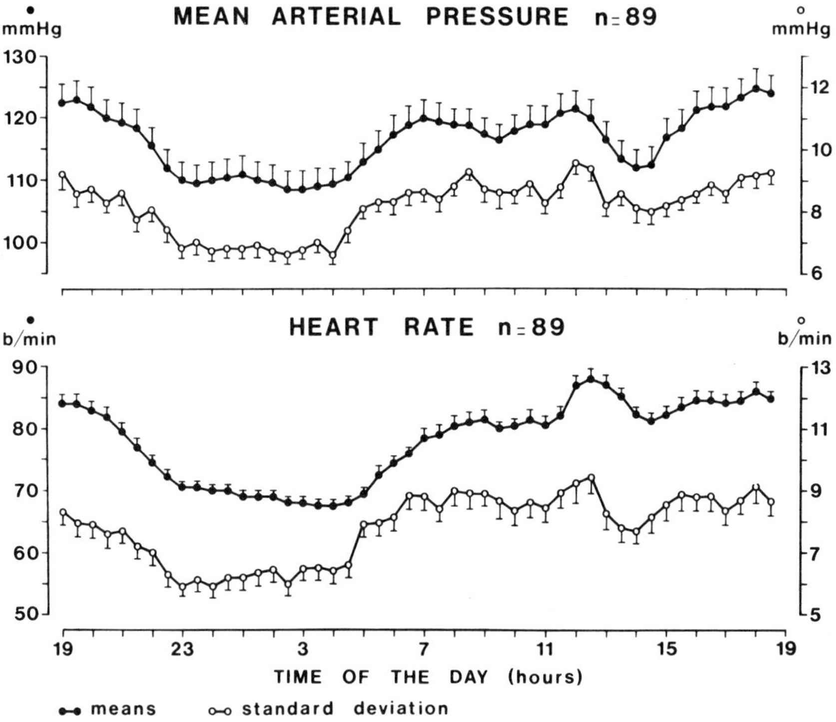

FIG. 3. The *black points* represent the mean arterial pressure and heart rate values separately obtained for the 48 half-hours of the recording. The *open circles* represent the corresponding absolute variabilities (standard deviations). The scale for the mean values is on the *left*, that for the variabilities on the *right*. Data are shown as means (±SE) of all 69 subjects. (From ref. 16, by permission.)

from normotensive to the most severe hypertensive patients (Fig. 4). Interestingly, borderline hypertensive patients are not characterized by any disproportionate increase in blood pressure variability, as formerly suggested by the term *labile hypertensives* proposed in the past (19). On the contrary, they exhibit blood pressure SDs that are just in between those of normotensive and mild hypertensive subjects. When blood pressure variability is expressed in percent, as a coefficient of variation, no more differences among different blood pressure groups are evident, however. Because the degree of blood pressure variability has been related to the effectiveness of neural control on the circulation, the similarity of normalized blood

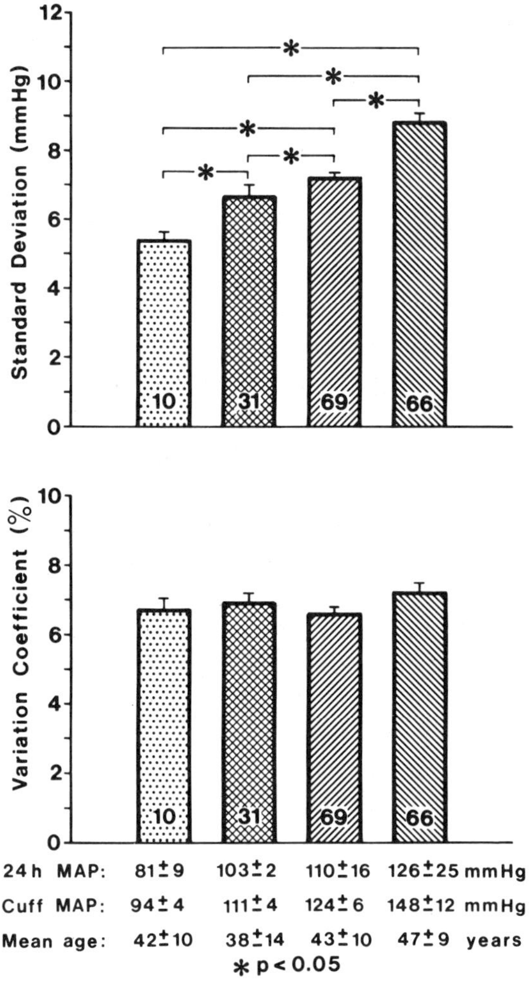

FIG. 4. Bar graphs of absolute (SD) and percent (varation coefficient) 24-hr variability of mean arterial blood pressure (MAP) in 10 normotensive, 31 borderline hypertensive, 69 moderately hypertensive, and 66 severe essential hypertensive subjects. Data are given as mean ± SEM for each group. *Asterisks* refer to statistical significance of between-group differences. (From ref. 6, by permission.)

pressure variability in subjects with normal and high blood pressure may suggest that hypertension is not associated with an impairment of mechanisms responsible for cardiovascular homeostasis.

Blood pressure variability, and particularly systolic blood pressure variability, increases also with age, at least when short-term blood pressure changes are considered, whereas heart rate variability decreases steadily with aging. These experimental findings account for the clinical impression of a greater blood pressure lability in the elderly, whereas the reduced heart rate variability in this age group may be due to the progressive reduction in the effectiveness of parasympathetic modulation of the heart, which is known to occur with aging (20).

FACTORS INVOLVED IN THE GENESIS OF BLOOD PRESSURE VARIATIONS

Behavioral Factors

Over 24 hr, blood pressure exhibits both rises and falls in response to different environmental stimuli of both physical or psychological nature. These changes may be of short duration, such as the blood pressure increases observed during exercise, exposure to cold, or public speaking (6). They may also last for hours, however, when the responsible stimulus is strong and/or persistent enough, as exemplified on the one hand by the prolonged increase in blood pressure observed in subjects playing cards or in university students undergoing examination (Fig. 5) and, on the other hand, by the steady reduction in blood pressure that characterizes sleep (6,18, 21–23) (Fig. 6). All these changes, which are paralleled by concordant changes in heart rate, are likely to be mediated mainly through influences originating in the central nervous system (6).

Role of Central and Reflex Neural Factors

Arterial baroreflexes are known to be involved in maintaining cardiovascular homeostasis. It is not surprising therefore that they have been shown to participate in modulating blood pressure variability. Direct evidence in this regard has been obtained in animals; in several species surgical baroreceptor deafferentation through sinoaortic denervation is associated with a consistent increase in blood

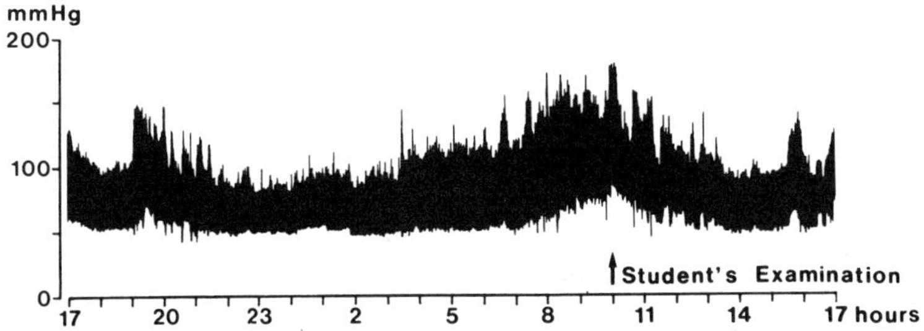

FIG. 5. A 24-hour intra-arterial blood pressure tracing performed in a medical student who at the time indicated by the *arrow* took an examination. The recording was started at 17.00 hours and ended at 17.00 hours on the following day.

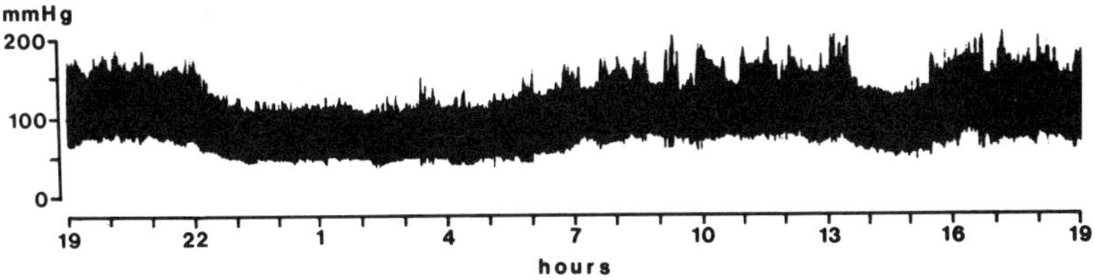

FIG. 6. A 24-hr intra-arterial blood pressure in a subject with untreated essential hypertension. Blood pressure was recorded by the Oxford method while the subject was hospitalized for a clinical evaluation of his hypertensive condition. During the recording the subject was left free to move within the hospital area and to live the social life of ambulant inpatients. There was a prolonged and marked fall in blood pressure during the night and an afternoon nap and short-term blood pressure rises during the day. (From ref. 67, by permission.)

pressure variability (24–28) (Fig. 7). In humans, similarly direct evidence is lacking. Only a few reports on the occurrence of a greater magnitude of blood pressure fluctuations in subjects with surgically denervated carotid sinuses are available (29,30). The influence on blood pressure variability exerted by arterial baroreflexes has been investigated in humans mainly in an indirect fashion (31–33). Information on this issue has been obtained by relating the degree of blood pressure variations to the sensitivity of the reflex control exerted by arterial baroreceptors on blood pressure and heart rate as assessed through a number of laboratory techniques (neck chamber manipulation of carotid baroreceptors, stimulation or deac-

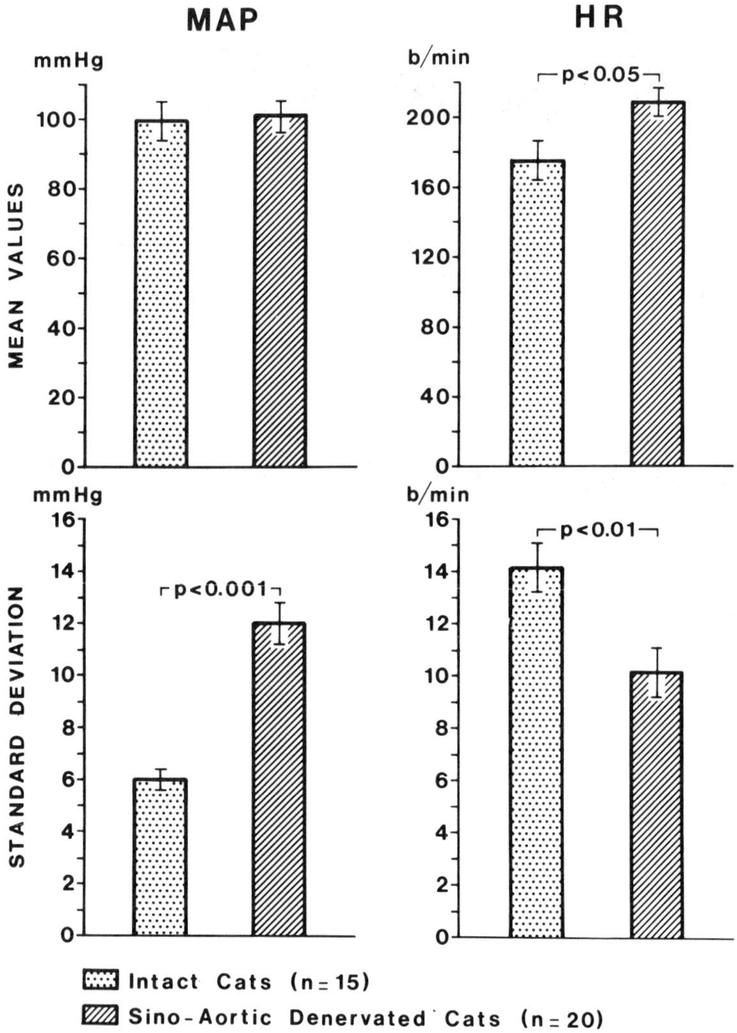

FIG. 7. Mean arterial pressure (MAP) and heart rate (HR) and their variabilities (coefficients of variation) in 15 intact cats and in 20 cats after sinoaortic denervation. Data are shown as means ± SE. (From ref. 28, by permission.)

tivation of arterial baroreceptors via intravenous injection of vasoactive drugs, etc.) (6).

Studies that have combined the above-mentioned laboratory techniques with ambulatory intra-arterial blood pressure monitoring have shown that blood pressure variability either long- or short-term, is inversely related to the sensitivity of arterial baroreceptor control of circulation (Fig. 8). In contrast, the sensitivity of these reflex mechanisms is directly related to the degree of heart rate variability over 24 hr. This may suggest that changes in heart rate, and thus in cardiac output, are instrumentally used by arterial baroreceptors to buffer the changes in blood pressure, no matter how the latter are induced. Although evident and statistically significant, the influence of baroreflex mechanisms on blood pressure and heart rate variability is not predominant, however, as demonstrated by the limited value of correlation coefficients between these phenomena. Actually, according to data from our group, no more than 25% of the between-subject difference in blood pressure variability can be accounted for by differences in baroreceptor reflex sensitivity (33). It is therefore likely that other factors besides baroreflexes play a major role in this regard. The above-mentioned parallelism that characterizes half-hour blood pressure and heart rate changes over 24 hr and the absence of a clear cause-and-effect relationship between blood pressure and heart rate changes demonstrated in both human and animal studies (34,35) suggest that blood pressure and heart rate changes over a 24-hr period are mainly modulated by influences that act on the heart and the peripheral circulation in a parallel fashion. As suggested also by the effects of behavior on circulation (see above), it is likely that these predominant influences come from the central nervous system, although other studies are needed to further clarify this issue (6,16,18).

Mechanical and Humoral Factors

Changes in blood pressure are also determined by the mechanics of ventilation (36), a factor that may contribute to blood pressure rhythmic oscillations within the frequency range of respiratory activity. Several reports have suggested the influence of humoral sub-

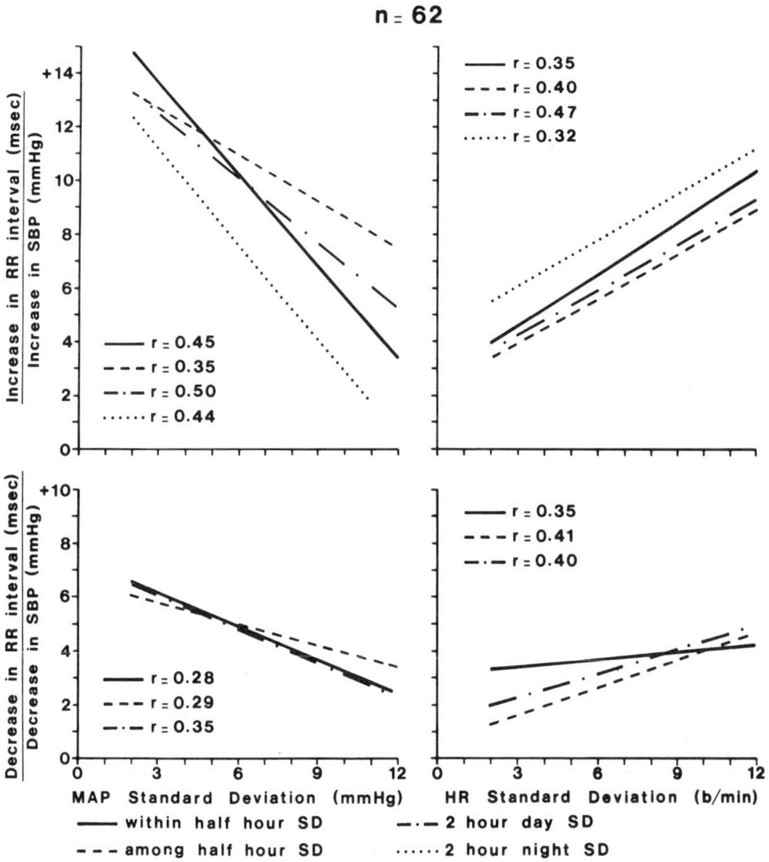

FIG. 8. Inverse relationship between 24-hr blood pressure variability and baroreflex sensitivity (*left panels*) and direct relationship between 24-hr heart rate variability and baroreflex sensitivity (*right panels*) in 62 subjects with untreated essential hypertension. Blood pressure and heart rate variability were obtained by calculating the standard deviation of the daytime mean arterial pressure and heart rate values, the nighttime arterial pressure and heart rate values, the average of the standard deviations of the 48 different half-hours in the recording period (standard deviation within half-hours) and the standard deviation obtained by averaging the 48 mean half-hour values (standard deviation among half-hours). Baroreflex sensitivity was assessed by calculating the slope of the linear regression between the lengthening of pulse interval induced by a phenylephrine-dependent rise in systolic blood pressure (SBP) or the shortening in the pulse interval induced by a trinitroglycerine-dependent fall in systolic blood pressure. (From ref. 31, by permission.)

stances on blood pressure variations over 24 hr. Plasma catecholamines are known to be responsible for the blood pressure peaks observed in patients with pheochromocytoma (37). Other hormones produced by the adrenal cortex may influence blood pressure changes, particularly in pathological conditions, as demonstrated by the alteration in the sleep-wakefulness cycle of blood pressure observed in patients with Cushing's syndrome or with hyperaldosteronism, although the latter finding is still a matter of debate (38,39). More generally, the renin-angiotensin system has been suggested to play some role in influencing blood pressure variability (40). Very little information is available on the possible effects of other humoral factors, such as vasopressin, atrial natriuretic factor (ANF), growth hormone (GH), sexual hormones, prostaglandins, etc. on blood pressure variability phenomena.

Blood Pressure "Rhythms"

As previously mentioned, blood pressure variability is characterized not only be erratic transient changes but also by rhythmic fluctuations, which recently have been shown to occur not only in standardized resting conditions but also throughout a dynamic 24-hr recording (17,41–44). The period of these fluctuations may range from few seconds, such as those associated with respiration, to 2 hours or even days or months. The latter include seasonal variations in blood pressure, the day-night blood pressure cycle, and other fluctuations in blood pressure lasting hours or minutes that can be variably observed over a 24-hr period. These rhythms may have different origins. It is still widely debated whether they are determined by one or several different inner "clocks" or, in contrast, represent the results of a complex interplay between the effects of internal "oscillators," behavioral activities, and periodic events such as respiration and the influences of a number of feedback regulatory mechanisms (42,45) acting through autonomic nervous system pathways on spontaneously contracting peripheral vascular smooth muscle cells.

All these mechanisms may be variably important in determining different "rhythms." For instance, it is quite unlikely that the day-night cycle of blood pressure may result only from an inner "circadian" rhythm as formerly suggested (46). On the contrary, there is evidence in favor of a major involvement of behavioral activities in modulating the sleep-wakefulness cycle of blood pressure. This hypothesis is supported by the observations on the reversal of the day-night changes in blood pressure and heart rate observed in shift workers (47,48). Faster blood pressure and heart rate rhythms, however, such as those having a frequency near 0.1 and 0.3 Hz, seem to be more clearly under the oscillating modulation of autonomic sympathetic and/or parasympathetic influences (41,49,50), although the modality of this modulation and its interference with other non-neural factors, such as the mechanical effects of respiration, still warrant further investigation.

BLOOD PRESSURE VARIABILITY: SCIENTIFIC APPLICATIONS

With the background of the above-mentioned experimental evidence provided by both animal and human studies, blood pressure variability can be taken as an index of the effectiveness of neural cardiovascular regulation. Thus, its dynamic analysis might represent a powerful tool to shed light on the features of this control in normal and pathological conditions throughout a 24-hr period. Two specific components of blood pressure and heart rate variability have been more deeply investigated in this regard: (a) the sequences of consecutive heart beats characterized by spontaneously occurring changes in blood pressure and by reflex reciprocal changes in heart rate, and (b) the rhythmic oscillations of blood pressure and heart rate at frequencies ranging between 0.025 and 0.5 Hz.

The Sequence Analysis Method

The analysis of the transient increases and reductions in blood pressure associated with reciprocal changes in heart rate that spontaneously take place over a 24-hr period has been proposed as a means to obtain dynamic information on baroreceptor modulation of the heart (17,51,52). By beat-to-beat computer analysis of a 24-hr recording, it is possible to automatically detect sequences of consecutive heartbeats characterized by hypertension/bradycardia and/or by hypotension/tachycardia. By analogy with the vasoactive drug injection technique (53), the calculation of the slope of the regression line between spontaneous changes in systolic blood pressure and reflex reciprocal changes in heart rate (expressed as changes in heart interval) can provide a quantitative index of the sensitivity of baroreceptor reflex control of heart rate (Fig. 9). The advantage of this method, as compared to the laboratory approach, is that the evaluation is obtained without external intervention on the cardiovascular system. More importantly, it can be carried out dynamically over the various behavioral conditions of daily life, not in an artificial laboratory environment. That these sequences are actually the results of the involvement of arterial baroreceptors in reflex control of the heart was demonstrated in the experimental animal by observing the almost complete disappearance of these transient events following baroreceptor denervation (51). Application of this method to humans, by computer analysis of 24-hr intra-arterial blood pressure recording (52), has shown that (a) the sensitivity of baroreceptor control of the heart is widely variable over 24 hr, being greater during the night and lower during the day; and (b) these sequences are less frequent and their slope is reduced in essential hypertension, where the nocturnal increase in baroreceptor sensitivity observed in normotensive subjects is not apparent (Fig. 10).

Spectral Analysis of Blood Pressure Rhythms

The existence of rhythmic oscillations in blood pressure and heart rate was described a long time ago (42). Only recently, however, have these rhythmic events been proposed as a means to reflect the features of autonomic regulation of the cardiovascular system (15, 41,44). Using power spectral analysis, three oscillations have been more frequently addressed in this context, occurring respectively at

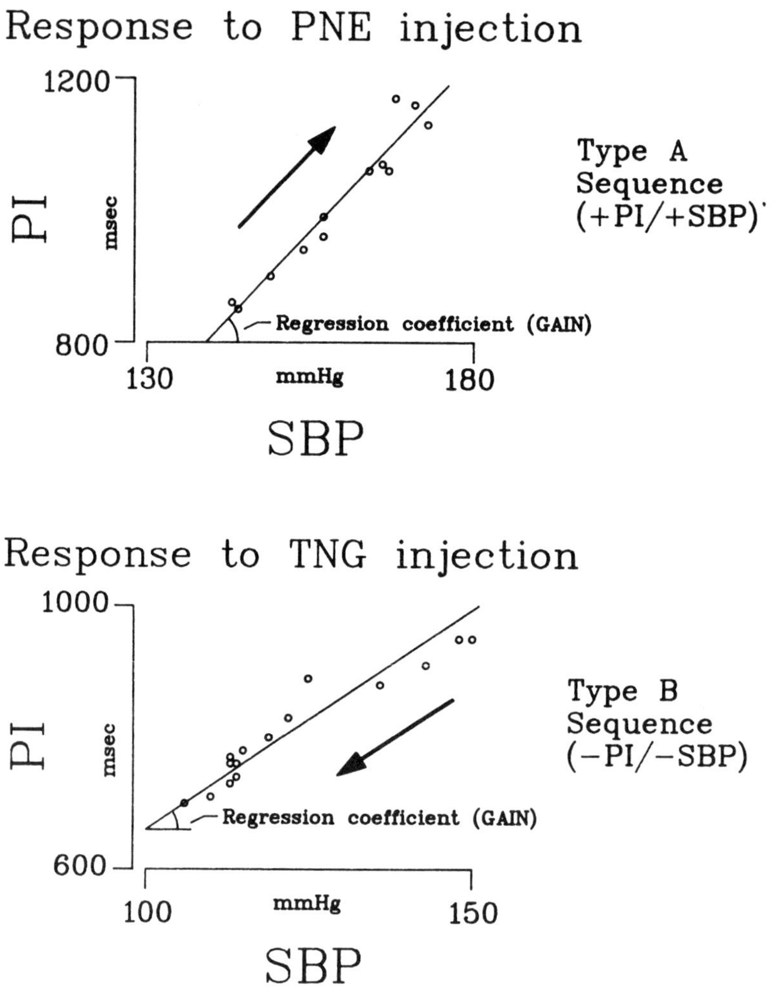

FIG. 9. This drawing illustrates how the spontaneously occurring hypertension/bradycardia (progressive increase in SBP and progressive lengthening in PI over consecutive beats) and hypotension/tachycardia (progressive reduction in SBP and progressive shortening in PI over consecutive beats) sequences were selected by the computer. The slope of the regression line between changes in SBP and changes in PI, when the correlation coefficient between the two sets of variable was $>.85$, was taken as an index of the sensitivity of baroreflex control of heart rate, similarly to the procedure adopted for the laboratory techniques based on injection of vasoactive drugs. PNE, phenylephine; TNG, nitroglycerin.

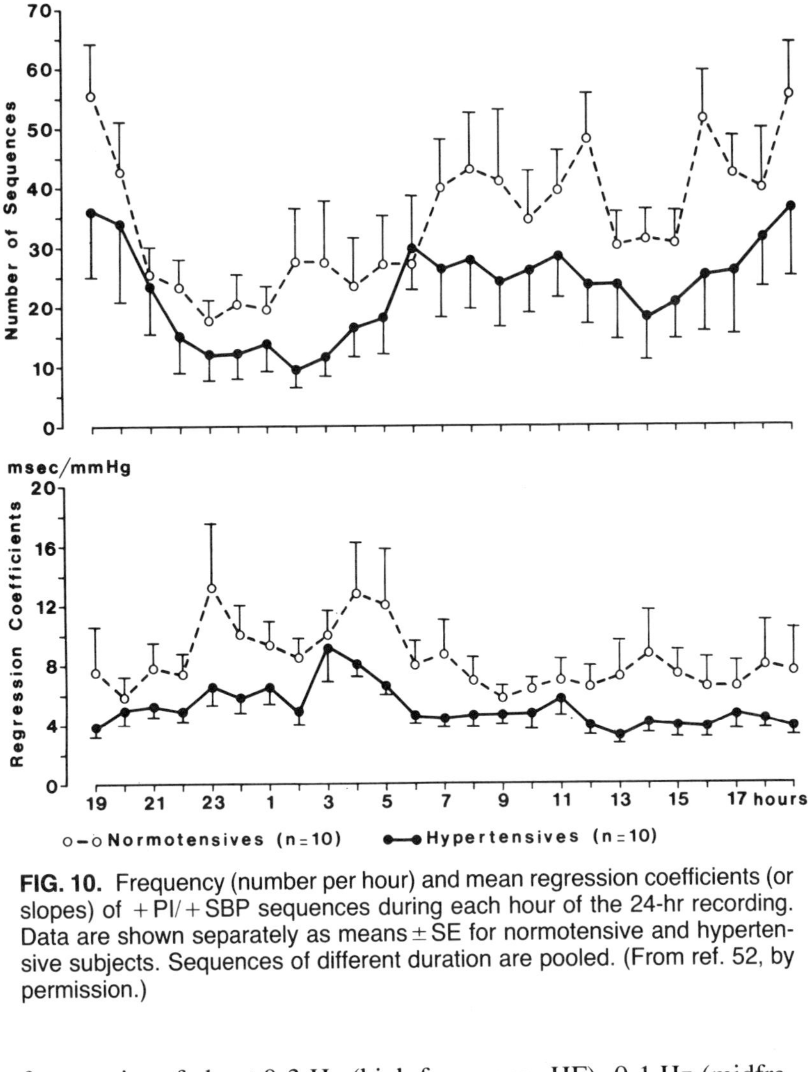

FIG. 10. Frequency (number per hour) and mean regression coefficients (or slopes) of +PI/+SBP sequences during each hour of the 24-hr recording. Data are shown separately as means ± SE for normotensive and hypertensive subjects. Sequences of different duration are pooled. (From ref. 52, by permission.)

frequencies of about 0.3 Hz (high frequency, HF), 0.1 Hz (midfrequency, MF) and 0.03 Hz (low frequency, LF) (Fig. 11). The power of HF oscillation has been suggested as reflecting respiratory modulated parasympathetic regulation of heart rate and mechanically induced blood pressure fluctuations synchronous with respiration (41,44,45,54,55). The power of MF oscillations has been proposed as reflecting parasympathetic and sympathetic modulation of

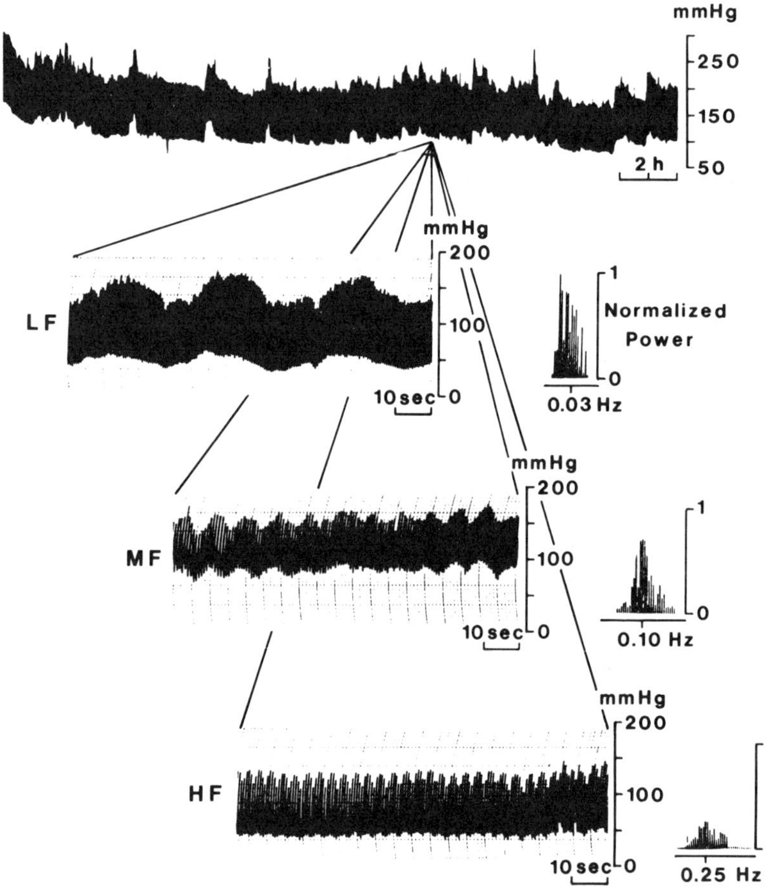

FIG. 11. A 24-hour intra-arterial tracing showing blood pressure oscillations with different period. Examples of blood pressure oscillations at different frequency are also shown. LF, low frequency oscillations with a period of 30 sec (0.03 Hz); MF, midfrequency oscillations with a period of 10 sec (0.1 Hz); HF, high frequency oscillations with a period of 5 sec (0.25 Hz).

heart rate, sympathetic regulation of vasomotor tone, and a possible resonance in the arterial baroreflex loop (44,45,56,57). Still unknown is the physiologic meaning of LF blood pressure and heart rate oscillations, although there are suggestions on their possible relationship with thermoregulatory mechanisms involved in the modulation of peripheral vessels or with the influences on circulation exerted by the renin-angiotensin system (58,59).

We have recently shown that it is possible to carry out a dynamic spectral analysis of these phenomena throughout 24 hr (17,43), and we have demonstrated the existence of a day-night modulation of these rhythmic events, too. The most striking changes are the nighttime reduction in MF powers of blood pressure and the nighttime increase in HF powers of heart rate (Fig. 12). These changes may reflect the reduction in sympathetic activity and the simultaneous increase in parasympathetic activity, which is known to occur during sleep (60), but they may also be importantly affected by different respiratory patterns between daytime activities and sleep. Further information can be obtained by computing the ratio between the spectral powers of systolic blood pressure and pulse interval (the reciprocal of heart rate) in the frequency bands where these two signals are highly coherent, that is near 0.1 and 0.3 Hz. This ratio has been proposed as an additional means to quantify baroreflex control of heart rate (15,61,62) from spontaneously occurring blood pressure and heart rate changes.

Thus, both the sequence analysis and power spectrum analysis of rhythmic blood pressure and heart rate events represent new and promising approaches to the dynamic evaluation of the mechanisms involved in cardiovascular regulation. These techniques may find important applications in healthy subjects and in disease conditions (63–66).

BLOOD PRESSURE VARIABILITY: CLINICAL RELEVANCE

As already suggested by Riva-Rocci, the fact that blood pressure is characterized by continuous changes also has important clinical implications. First, the occurrence of marked and unpredictable rises in blood pressure at the time of office blood pressure measurements is relevant both from the diagnostic and prognostic point of view (67–69). This emotionally induced pressor reaction may be important insofar as it may introduce an error of overestimation in the diagnosis of a hypertensive condition (70,71). On the other hand, it has also been suggested that the occurrence of this "white-coat" hypertension may itself imply negative prognostic implica-

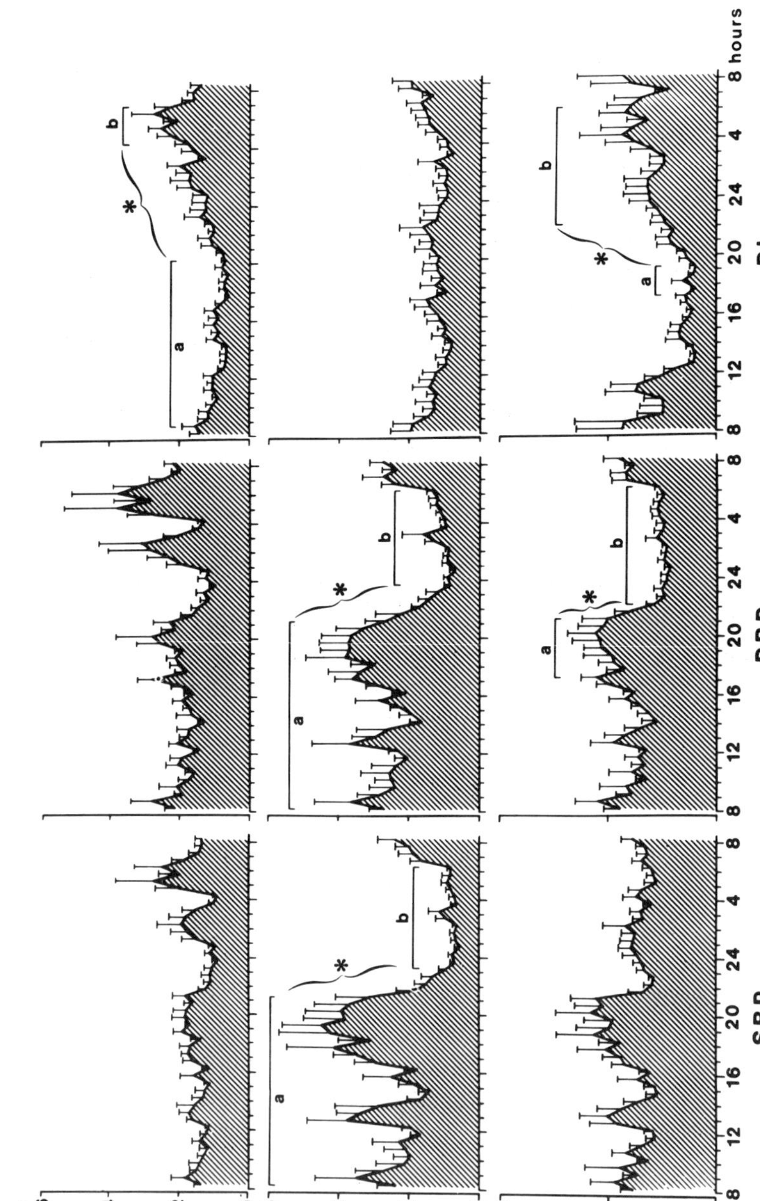

LF
MF
HF
%
SBP
DBP
PI
8 hours
n = 10
* p < 0.02

tions, because subjects characterized by this reaction share several features with people having sustained arterial hypertension (72). This uncertainty on the clinical interpretation of the "white-coat" phenomenon could be clarified only by means of prospective morbidity and mortality studies, which are presently lacking.

Second, studies that have related the degree of 24-hr blood pressure variability to the rate of cardiovascular complications of hypertension have suggested that the occurrence of frequent blood pressure peaks over the day and night bears a relationship with the frequency and the severity of target organ damage of hypertension (73,74). According to the results of these investigations, people with comparable 24-hr blood pressure levels may have more or less target organ damage as a function of the degree of their blood pressure variability, expressed as the 24-hr standard deviation (Fig. 13). Even if this suggestion also needs to be confirmed by prospective studies, these preliminary observations nevertheless underline the potential diagnostic relevance of blood pressure variability phenomena as early markers of possible cardiovascular complications.

Third, due to the relationship between blood pressure fluctuations and the effectiveness of the mechanisms responsible for cardiovascular homeostasis, the assessment of blood pressure variability may also be important in the diagnosis of alterations in neural autonomic regulation of the cardiovascular system, which may characterize diabetes, uremia, heart failure, acute myocardial infarction (AMI), essential dysautonomia, etc. (6,64,75–80). The degree of blood pressure variability over 24 hr or in the daytime has also been proposed as an index of the sympathetic mediated cardiovascular reactivity to daily life stress. This approach might overcome some limitations of traditional laboratory stressors in assessing subjects' reactivity to stress (81–83), but its routine use in this field is made

FIG. 12. Graphs showing low- (LF), mid- (MF), and high- (HF) frequency powers of systolic blood pressure (SBP), diastolic blood pressure (DBP), and pulse interval (PI) for 10 mild essential hypertensive subjects. Data are averaged for each half-hour and shown as mean ± SEM. Powers are represented as percent of 24-hr variance. *Asterisks* refer to statistical significance of difference between subperiods of day (*a*) and night (*b*). Subperiod duration is indicated by *horizontal bars*. (From ref. 17, by permission.)

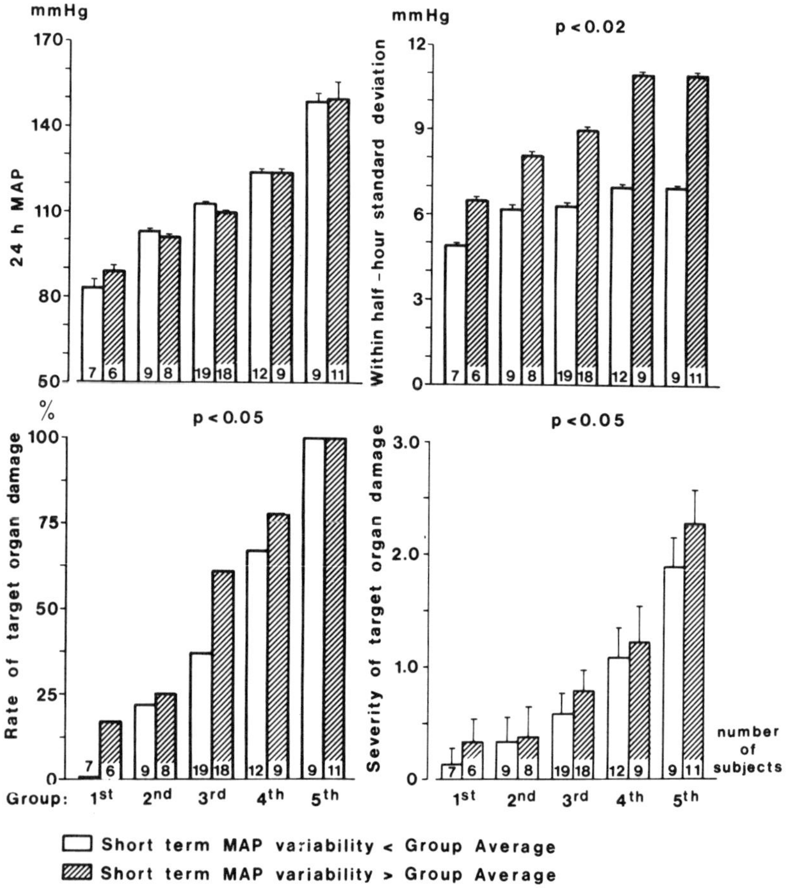

FIG. 13. Rate and severity of target organ damage in 108 patients. The patients were divided into five groups according to the increasing value of their 24-hr MAP. Within each 24-hr MAP group, the patients were further subdivided into two classes according to whether their short-term blood pressure variability, expressed as within half-hour standard deviation of MAP, was below or above the average short-term variability of the group. Note that within each group the two classes had a similar 24-hr MAP, but that the rate and the severity of target organ damage was less in the class in which blood pressure variability was lower. (From ref. 73, by permission.)

difficult by the somewhat anecdotal nature of blood pressure and heart rate responses to behavioral stress and by the related difficulty in providing "normal" standards (83).

Finally, the assessment of 24-hr blood pressure variability may also provide important information in clinical pharmacology, to exclude possible effects of antihypertensive drugs on cardiovascular homeostasis. According to presently available evidence, gathered by means of a 24-hr ambulatory blood pressure monitoring (ABPM), most antihypertensive agents reduce the 24-hr SD. This reduction, however, is proportional to the reduction in 24-hr blood pressure mean values, so that percent measures of blood pressure variability (coefficient of variation) are not affected. This may suggest that most drugs currently employed to treat hypertensive patients can be considered safe in this regard (6,84–88).

CONCLUSIONS

The availability in recent years of techniques for ambulatory blood pressure monitoring has facilitated obtaining a more detailed picture of blood pressure variability over 24 hr. The analysis of beat-to-beat blood pressure recordings obtained in daily life conditions has provided a deeper insight into the different components that contribute to the blood pressure variations occurring in every period of the day and the night. This has offered new perspectives for both pathophysiologic investigations of neural cardiovascular control mechanisms and the diagnostic and, it is hoped, prognostic evaluation of hypertensive patients. The development of new techniques for monitoring beat-to-beat blood pressure noninvasively in ambulatory subjects will extend the feasibility of studies on blood pressure variability over a broader range of physiologic and pathologic conditions where intra-arterial recordings cannot be easily performed.

REFERENCES

1. Hales S. Statistical essays. In: Innys, Mauby, eds. *Haemastaticks*, vol 2. 1733.
2. Marey EJ. Recherches sur l'tat de la circulation d'aprs les caractres du pouls, fournis par un nouveau sphymographe. In: *Gazette hebdomadaire de medecine et chirurgie*, vol 7. Paris: Masson, 1860.

3. Ozanam C. *La circulation et le pouls*. Paris: Librairie Boilire, 1886.
4. Riva-Rocci S. La tecnica della sfigmomanometria. *Gazz Med Torino* 1897; 10:181–191.
5. Mancia G. Methods for assessing blood pressure values in humans. *Hypertension* 1983;5:III-5.
6. Mancia G, Zanchetti A. Blood pressure variability. In: Zanchetti A, Tarazi R, eds. *Handbook of hypertension*, vol 7. Amsterdam: Elsevier, 1986;125–152.
7. Bevan AT, Honour AJ, Stott FH. Direct arterial pressure recording in unrestricted man. *Clin Sci* 1969;36:329.
8. Stott FH, Teny VG, Honour AJ. Factors determining the design and construction of a portable pressure transducer system. *Postgrad Med J* 1976;52(suppl 7):97–99.
9. Gould BA, Hornung RS, Cashman PM, Raftery EB. An evaluation of the Avionics Pressumeter III 1978 at home and in hospital. *Clin Cardiol* 1986; 9:335–343.
10. Casadei R, Parati G, Pomidossi G, Groppelli A, Trazzi S, Mancia G. 24 hour blood pressure monitoring: evaluation of Spacelabs 5300 Monitor by comparison with intra-arterial blood pressure recording in ambulant subjects. *J Hypertens* 1988;6:797–803.
11. Di Rienzo M, Grassi G, Pedotti A, Mancia G. Continuous vs intermittent blood pressure measurements in estimating 24 hour average blood pressure. *Hypertension* 1983;5:264–266.
12. Wesseling KH, De Wit B, Settels JJ, Klawer WH. On the indirect registration of finger blood pressure after Peñaz. *Funkt Biol Med* 1982;1:245–250.
13. Parati G, Casadei R, Groppelli A, Di Rienzo M, Mancia G. Comparison of finger and intra-arterial blood pressure monitoring at rest and during laboratory testing. *Hypertension* 1989;13:647–655.
14. Langewouters GJ, De Wit B, Van der Hoeven GMA, Van Montfrans GA, Imholz BPM, Wieling WW, Wesseling KH. Feasibility of continuous non invasive 24h ambulatory measurements of finger arterial blood pressure with Portapres. *J Hypertens* 1990;8(suppl 3):S88.
15. De Boer RW, Karemaker JM, Van Montfrans GA. Determination of baroreflex sensitivity by spectral analysis of spontaneous blood pressure and heart rate fluctuations in man. In: Lown B, Malliani A, Prosdocimi M, Eds. *Neural mechanisms and cardiovascular disease*, vol 5. Fidia Research Series, Liviana Press, 1986;303–315.
16. Mancia G, Ferrari A, Gregorini L, Bertinieri G, Grassi G, Parati G, Pomidossi G, Di Rienzo M, Pedotti A, Zanchetti A. Blood pressure and heart rate variability in normotensive and hypertensive human beings. *Circ Res* 1983;53:96–104.
17. Parati G, Castiglioni P, Di Rienzo M, Omboni S, Pedotti A, Mancia G. Sequential spectral analysis of 24 hour blood pressure and pulse interval in humans. *Hypertension* 1990;16:414–421.
18. Mancia G, Bertinieri G, Cavallazzi A, Di Rienzo M, Parati G, Pomidossi G, Ramirez AJ, Zanchetti A. Mechanisms of blood pressure variability in man. *Clin Exp Hypertens* 1985;A7:167.
19. Julius S, Ellis CN, Pasqual AV, Matice M, Hansson L, Hunyor SN, Sandler L. Home blood pressure determination: value in borderline (labile) hypertension. *JAMA* 1974;229:663.

20. Ferrari AJ, Grassi G, Mancia G. Alterations of reflex control in circulation with aging. In: Amery A, Staessen J, eds. Hypertension in the elderly. *Handbook of hypertension*, vol 12. Amsterdam: Elsevier, 1989;39–50.
21. Mancia G, Ferrari AU, Gregorini L, Parati G, Cioffi P, Di Rienzo M, Pedotti A. Continuous intra-arterial blood pressure recording in human hypertension. In: Sambhi M, ed. *The fundamental fault in hypertension*. The Haag: Martinus Nijhoff, 1984;235.
22. Littler WA, Honour AJ, Carter RD, Sleight P. Sleep and blood pressure. *Br Med J* 1975;3:346.
23. Pickering TG, Harshfield JA, Kleinert HD, Blank S, Laragh JH. Blood pressure during normal daily activities, sleep and exercise. *JAMA* 1982;247:992.
24. Cowley AW, Liard LF, Guyton AC. Role of the baroreceptor reflex in daily control of arterial blood pressure and other variables in dogs. *Circ Res* 1973; 32:564.
25. Norman NA, Coleman TG, Dent AC. Continuous monitoring of arterial pressure indicates sino-aortic denervated rats are not hypertensive. *Hypertension* 1981;3:119.
26. Krieger EM. Neurogenic hypertension in the rat. *Circ Res* 1964;15:511.
27. Ito Sker AM. Hypertension following denervation of aortic baroreceptor in unanesthetized dogs. *Circ Res* 1979;45:26.
28. Ramirez AJ, Bertinieri G, Belli L, Cavallazzi A, Di Rienzo M, Pedotti A, Mancia G. Reflex control of blood pressure and heart rate by arterial baroreceptors and by cardiopulmonary receptors in unanesthetized cat. *J Hypertens* 1985;3:327.
29. Riplay RC, Hollifield GW, Nies AS. Sustained hypertension after section of the glossopharyngeal nerve. *Am J Med* 1977;62:297.
30. Pessina A, Palatini P, Casiglia E, Sperti G, Mormino P, Di Marco A, Dal Palú C. Evaluation of blood pressure control after bilateral glomectomy: effects of propranolol treatment. In: Dal Palú C, Pessina A, eds. *ISAM 1985: Proceedings of the Vth International Symposium on Ambulatory Monitoring*. Padua: CLEUP, 1985;153.
31. Mancia G, Ferrari AU, Gregorini L, Parati G, Pomidossi G, Bertinieri G, Grassi G, Zanchetti A. Arterial pressure variability in man: its relation to high blood pressure, age and baroreflex sensitivity. *Clin Sci* 1980;59:401s–404s.
32. Conway J, Boon N, Davies C, Jones JV, Sleight P. Neural and humoral mechanisms involved in blood pressure variability. *J Hypertens* 1984;2:203.
33. Mancia G, Parati G, Pomidossi G, Casadei R, Di Rienzo M, Zanchetti A. Arterial baroreflexes and blood pressure and heart rate variabilities in humans. *Hypertension* 1986;8:147–153.
34. Parati G, Pomidossi G, Casadei R, Groppelli A, Trazzi S, Di Rienzo M, Mancia G. Role of heart rate variability in the production of blood pressure variability in man. *J Hypertens* 1987;5:557–560.
35. Ferrari AU, Daffonchio A, Albergati F, Mancia G. Inverse relationship between heart rate and blood pressure variability in rats. *Hypertension* 1987; 10:533–537.
36. Doenhorst AC, Howard P, Leathart GL. Respiratory variations in blood pressure. *Circulation* 1952;6:553–558.
37. Mancia G, Ferrari AU, Gregorini L, Parati G, Pomidossi G, Zanchetti A.

Prolonged intra-arterial blood pressure recording diagnosis of pheochromocitoma. *Lancet* 1979;2:1193–1194.

38. Imai Y, Abe K, Sasaki S, et al. Altered circadian blood pressure rhythm in patients with Cushing's syndrome. *Hypertension* 1988;12:11–19.
39. Imai Y, Munakata M, Abe K, Sekino K. The circadian blood pressure variation in patients with disturbance of renin-angiotensin-aldosterone system and with renal disease [in Japanese]. In: Koshikawa S, Nagasawa T, Koiso K, Ito H, eds. *Annual review of nephrology*. Tokyo: Chugaigakusha, 1990;141–151.
40. Watson RDS, Stallard TJ, Flinn RM, Littler WA. Factors determining pressure and its variability in hypertensive man. *Hypertension* 1980;2:333.
41. Akselrod S, Gordon D, Madwed JB, Snidmann NC, Shannon DC, Cohen RG. Hemodynamic regulation: investigation by spectral analysis. *Am J Physiol* 1985;249:H867–H875.
42. Koepchen HP. History of studies and concepts of blood pressure waves. In: Miyakawa K et al. eds. *Mechanisms of blood pressure waves*. Tokyo: Japan Sci Soc Press. Berlin: Springer-Verlag, 1984;3–23.
43. Di Rienzo M, Castiglioni P, Mancia G, Parati G, Pedotti A. 24-hour sequential spectral analysis of arterial blood pressure and pulse interval in free-moving subjects. *IEEE Trans Biomed Eng* 1989;36:1066–1074.
44. Furlan R, Guzzetti S, Crivellaro W, Dazzi S, Tinelli M, Baselli G, Cerutti S, Lombardi F, Pagani M, Malliani A. Continuous 24-hour assessment of the neural regulation of systemic arterial pressure and RR variabilities in ambulant subjects. *Circulation* 1990;81:537–547.
45. Saul JP, Albrecht P, Berger RD, Cohen RJ. Analysis of long term heart rate variability: methods, 1/f scaling and implications. *Comp Cardiol* 1988; 419–422.
46. Millar-Craig MW, Bishop CN, Raftery EB. Circadian variation of blood pressure. *Lancet* 1978;1:795.
47. Floras JS, Jones SV, Johnston JA, Brooks DE, Hassan MO, Sleight P. Arousal and the circadian rhythm of blood pressure. *Clin Sci Mol Med* 1978; 55:395S.
48. Sundberg S, Kohvakka A, Gordin A. Rapid reversal of circadian blood pressure rhythm in shift workers. *J Hypertens* 1988;5:393–396.
49. Pagani M, Lombardi F, Guzzetti S, Rimoldi O, Furlan R, Pizzinelli P, Sandroni G, Malfatto G, Dell'Orto S, Piccaluga E, Turiel M, Baselli G, Cerutti S, Malliani A. Power spectral analysis of heart rate and arterial pressure variabilities as a marker of sympatho-vagal interaction in man and conscious dog. *Circ Res* 1986;59:178–193.
50. Appel MI, Berger RD, Saul JP, Smith JM, Cohen RJ. Beat-to-beat variability in cardiovascular variables: noise or music? *J Am Coll Cardiol* 1989;14:1139–1148.
51. Bertinieri G, Di Rienzo M, Cavallazzi A, Ferrari AU, Pedotti A, Mancia G. Evaluation of baroreceptor reflex by blood pressure monitoring in unanesthetized cats. *Am J Physiol* 1988;254:H377–H383.
52. Parati G, Di Rienzo M, Bertinieri G, Pomidossi G, Casadei R, Groppelli A, Pedotti A, Zanchetti A, Mancia G. Evaluation of the baroreceptor-heart rate reflex by 24-hour intra-arterial blood pressure monitoring in humans. *Hypertension* 1988;12:214–222.
53. Smyth HS, Sleight P, Pickering GW. Reflex regulation of arterial pressure

during sleep in man: a quantitative method for assessing baroreflex sensitivity. *Cir Res* 1969;24:109–121.
54. Saul JP, Berger RD, Chen MH, Cohen R. Transfer function analysis of autonomic regulation. II. Respiratory sinus arhythmia. *Am J Physiol* 1989; 256:H153–H161.
55. Pomerance B, Macaulay RJB, Caudill MA, Kutr I, Adam D, Gordon D, Killborn KM, Barger AG, Shannon DC, Cohen RJ, Benson H. Assessment of autonomic function in humans by heart rate spectral analysis. *Am J Physiol* 1986;84:H151–H153.
56. Saul JP. Beat-to-beat variation of heart rate reflect modulation of cardiac autonomic outflow. *NIPS* 1990;32–37.
57. Saul JP, Rea RF, Eckberg DL, Berger RD, Cohen RJ. Heart rate and muscle sympathetic nerve variability during reflex changes of autonomic activity. *Am J Physiol* 1990;258:H713–H721.
58. Kitney RI. An analysis of the non linear behaviour of the human thermal vasomotor control system. *J Theor Biol* 1975;62:231–248.
59. Eliosh S, Cohen S, Akselrod S. The role of Renin-Angiotensin and alpha control in the regulation of blood pressure in normotensive versus a hypertensive system. *Comput Cardiol* 1990.
60. Mancia G, Zanchetti A. Cardiovascular regulation during sleep. In: Orem J, ed. *Physiology during sleep*. New York: Academic Press, 1980;1.
61. Robbe HWJ, Mulder LJM, Ruddel H, Langewitz WA, Veldman JBP, Mulder G. Assessment of baroreceptor reflex sensitivity by means of spectral analysis. *Hypertension* 1987;10:538–543.
62. Pagani M, Somers V, Furlan R, Dell'Orto S, Conway J, Baselli G, Cerutti S, Sleight P, Malliani A. Changes in autonomic regulation induced by physical training in mild hypertension. *Hypertension* 1988;12(6):600–610.
63. Pagani M, Malfatto G, Pierini S, Casati R, Masu AM, Poli M, Guzzetti S, Lombardi F, Cerutti S, Malliani A. Power spectral analysis of the heart rate variability in the assessment of autonomic diabetic neuropathy. *J Auton Nerv Syst* 1988;23:143–153.
64. Saul PJ, Arai Y, Berger RD, Lilly LS, Colucci WS, Cohen RJ. Assessment of autonomic regulation in chronic congestive heart failure by heart rate spectral analysis. *Am J Cardiol* 1988;61:1292–1299.
65. Sands KEF, Appel ML, Lilly LS, Schoen FG, Mudge GM, Cohen RJ. Power spectrum analysis of heart rate variability in human cardiac transplant recipients. *Circulation* 1989;79:76–82.
66. Gordon D, Herrera VL, McAlpine L, Cohen R, Akselrod SL, Lang P, Norwood WI. Heart rate spectral analysis: a non invasive probe of cardiovascular regulation in initially ill children with heart disease. *Pediatr Cardiol* 1988; 9:69–74.
67. Mancia G. Ambulatory blood pressure monitoring in hypertension research and clinical practice. In: *Hypertension Yearbook, 1986*. International Society of Hypertension; Gower Academic Journals, 1986;93–116.
68. Parati G, Mutti E, Ravogli A, Trazzi S, Villani A, Mancia G. Advantages and disadvantages of non-invasive ambulatory blood pressure monitoring. *J Hypertens* 1990;8(suppl 6):S33–S38.
69. Mancia G, Parati G. Experience with 24-hour ambulatory blood pressure monitoring in hypertension. *Am Heart J* 1988;116:1134–1140.

70. Mancia G, Bertinieri G, Parati G, Pomidossi G, Ferrari AU, Gregorini L, Zanchetti A. Effects of blood pressure measurements by the doctor on patient's blood pressure and heart rate. *Lancet* 1983;2:695–698.
71. Mancia G, Parati G, Pomidossi G, Grassi G, Casadei R, Zanchetti A. Alerting reaction and rise in blood pressure during measurement by physician and nurse. *Hypertension* 1987;9:209–215.
72. Julius S, Mejia A, Jones K, Krause L, Schork N, van de Ven C, Johnson E, Petrin J, Sekkarie MA, Kjeldsen SE, Schmoulder R, Gupta R, Ferraro J, Nazzaro P, Weissfeld J. "White coat" versus "sustained" borderline hypertension in Tecumseh, Michigan. *Hypertension* 1990;16:617–623.
73. Parati G, Pomidossi G, Albini F, Malaspina D, Mancia G. Relationship of 24-hour blood pressure mean and variability to severity of target organ damage in hypertension. *J Hypertens* 1987;5:93–98.
74. Pessina AC, Palatini P, Sperti G, Cordoni L, Libardoni M, Mos L, Mormino PM, Di Marco A, Dal Palú C. Evaluation of hypertension and related target organ damage by average day-time blood pressure. *Clin Exp Hypertens* 1985; A7:267.
75. Ewing DJ, Campbell IW, Clarke BF. Assessment of cardiovascular effects in diabetic. *Ann Intern Med* 1980;7:308–311.
76. Grassi G, Parati G, Pomidossi G, Giannattasio C, Casadei R, Bolla G, Saino A, Casati S, Graziani G, Mancia G. Effects of haemodialysis and kidney transplantation on carotid and cardiopulmonary baroreflexes in uremic patients. *J Hypertens* 1987;5(suppl 5):S367–S369.
77. Kleiger RE, Miller JP, Bigger JT, Moss AJ. Decreased heart rate variability and its association with increased morbidity after acute myocadrial infarction. *Am J Cardiol* 1987;59:256–282.
78. Osculati G, Grassi G, Giannattasio C, Serravalle G, Valagussa F, Zanchetti A, Mancia G. Early alteration of baroreceptor control of heart rate in patients with acute myocardial infarction. *Circulation* 1990;81:939–948.
79. Schwartz PJ, Stone HL. The role of the autonomic nervous system in sudden coronary death. *Ann NY Acad Sci* 1982;382:162–181.
80. Shy GM, Drager GA. A neurological syndrome associated with orthostatic hypotension. *Arch Neurol* 1960;2:511–527.
81. Parati G, Pomidossi G, Ramirez AJ, Cesana B, Mancia G. Variability of the haemodynamic responses to laboratory tests employed in assessment of neural cardiovascular regulation in man. *Clin Sci* 1985;69:533–540.
82. Parati G, Pomidossi G, Casadei R, Ravogli A, Groppelli A, Cesana B, Mancia G. Comparison of the cardiovascular effects of different laboratory stressors and their relationship with blood pressure variability. *J Hypertens* 1988;6:481–488.
83. Mancia G, Parati G. Reactivity to physical and behavioral stress and blood pressure variability in hypertension. In: Julius S, Basset DR, eds. *Handbook of hypertension*, New York: Elsevier, 1987;104–122.
84. Mancia G, Pomidossi G, Parati G, Bertinieri G, Grassi G, Navone F, Ferrari AU, Gregorini L, Zanchetti A. Blood pressure response to labetalol in twice and three times daily administration during a 24-hour period. *Br J Clin Pharmacol* 1982;13:27S.
85. Pomidossi G, Parati G, Malaspina D, Camesasca C, Motolese M, Mancia G, Zanchetti A. Antihypertensive effect of a new formulation of slow release oxprenolol in essential hypertension. *Cardiovasc Pharmacol* 1987;10:593–598.

86. Mancia G, Ferrari AU, Pomidossi G, Parati G, Bertinieri G, Grassi G, Gregorini L, Zanchetti A. 24-hour hemodynamic profile during treatment of essential hypertension with once-a-day nadolol. *Hypertension* 1983;5:573.
87. Parati G, Pomidossi G, Casadei R, Trazzi S, Ravogli S, Zanchetti A, Mancia G. Evaluation of the antihypertensive effect of celiprolol by ambulatory blood pressure monitoring. *Am J Cardiol* 1988;61:27C–33C.
88. Mancia G, Parati G, Pomidossi G, Colombo A, Cuspidi C, Lattuada S, Antivalle M, Rindi M, Libretti A, Botta G, Zanchetti A. Evaluation of the antihypertensive effect of once a day captopril by 24 hour ambulatory blood pressure monitoring. *J Hypertens* 1987;5(suppl 5):S591–S593.

Ambulatory Blood Pressure Recording,
edited by H. Brunner and B. Waeber.
Raven Press, Ltd., New York © 1992.

5

Borderline Hypertension

Michael A. Weber, Joel M. Neutel, David H. G. Smith,
Deanna G. Cheung, and William F. Graettinger

Veterans Administration Medical Center, Long Beach, California 90822, and the University of California, Irvine, California 92717

Hypertension is a common condition. Based on the diagnostic criteria recommended by the Joint National Committee on Detection, Evaluation, and Treatment of High Blood Pressure (1), over 20% of the adult population of the United States and other western countries is hypertensive. Not surprisingly, a majority of these patients have untreated blood pressure values that fall into a range usually classified as mild hypertension. The reliability of measurements in patients at the borderline of this diagnosis can be critical, for potential variations of only a few mmHg can influence the decision of whether or not treatment is appropriate.

The use of automated whole-day blood pressure monitoring equipment should be of considerable value in these patients. Reports from several investigators have described the alerting reaction or the phenomenon of "white-coat" hypertension in which patients are hypertensive in the medical office or clinic but have normal blood pressures elsewhere. The ability of ambulatory blood pressure monitoring to provide blood pressure data throughout the day makes it possible to decide if the conventionally obtained blood pressure readings are typical. An important factor adding to the feasibility of this testing has been the continued technical improvement of the monitoring devices. Although the early methods depended upon intra-arterial measurements, noninvasive methods have now become standard for diagnostic purposes. Modern equipment is compact, lightweight, and easily portable. Moreover, such early problems as noise and vibration have largely been eliminated.

THE PROBLEM OF BORDERLINE HYPERTENSION: WHO SHOULD BE TREATED?

Clearly there is no difficulty in deciding upon treatment in patients with moderate to severe hypertension, for it has been well established that their high incidence of serious cardiovascular complications can be reduced markedly by antihypertensive therapy (2). It is also accepted that mild hypertension increases the probability of cardiovascular events, but the benefits of treatment for this large subgroup of patients have been less well defined. Both the Medical Research Council Trial (3) and the Australian Therapeutic Trial in Mild Hypertension (4) demonstrated that patients treated for mild hypertension had a lower incidence of major complications, especially strokes, than patients receiving placebo. But the cost of these benefits was high. It was estimated that the prevention of one major event in the Medical Research Council Trial (3) required the equivalent of 800 patient years of treatment. A reason for this finding was that the incidence of major events in the placebo-treated group was low, making it difficult to show a clear advantage for patients receiving active treatment. Thus, despite the actuarial risk apparently associated with mild hypertension, the majority of individual patients in short-term formal trials do not display a susceptibility to cardiovascular disease. One explanation for the unexpectedly good outcome in the placebo group came from the Australian Therapeutic Trial (4), where it was observed that over 40% of placebo-treated patients had clearly lower blood pressures after 3 or 4 years of observation than at baseline. Indeed, approximately 20% of the placebo-treated patients finished the trial with normal blood pressures. This phenomenon also has been observed in other therapeutic trials (5,6). The high placebo response rates occurred despite rigorous attempts to establish the diagnosis of hypertension by repeated blood pressure measurements during several weeks of pretrial placebo administration. These experiences support the conclusions of other investigators that the problem of "white-coat" hypertension cannot easily be solved by multiple measurements during a short period of time (7), but instead may take months or years to establish when conventional blood pressure measurements are employed.

The best basis for these findings is that many of the patients entering the hypertension clinical trials actually were normotensive, despite the care with which they were initially evaluated. This also may be the explanation why some patients discontinued from antihypertensive therapy may remain normotensive on an indefinite basis (8). There appear to be two principal solutions to the problem of overdiagnosis and inappropriate treatment: first, to improve the quality of the overall clinical assessment, and second, to improve diagnostic accuracy by using automated blood pressure monitoring procedures.

The Clinical Approach

The consideration of clinical factors that can influence the decision of whether to treat mild hypertension is, in reality, the complement of the indication for performing blood pressure monitoring. Thus, the indication for performing this procedure is the absence of clinical factors that would normally compel treatment. In patients with borderline or mild hypertension, the most important stimulus for initiating therapy is the presence of concurrent cardiovascular risk factors. Data from epidemiologic surveys have indicated that the presence of hypercholesterolemia or cigarette smoking strongly exaggerates the likelihood of complications, even when the hypertension is mild. Beyond the epidemiologic associations, it has been suggested that hypertensive vascular smooth muscle may bind with extra avidity to low density lipoproteins (9). Moreover, clinical studies have indicated that decreases in coronary events are far greater when both the hypertension and lipid problems are addressed concurrently (10). The presence of diabetes mellitus also acts as a spur to treatment of hypertension (11). Similarly, evidence for renal insufficiency or even minor degrees of proteinuria justify immediate treatment of hypertension. The prognosis of patients in whom there is already evidence for such cardiac changes as left ventricular hypertrophy or ischemic heart disease tends to be poor and usually necessitates the treatment of hypertension. Beyond these findings of concurrent risk factors, or of evidence for ongoing cardiovascular changes, the presence of a family history of hyper tension or premature cardiovascular disease further simplifies the course of action in patients with borderline hypertension.

Thus, many patients with modestly increased blood pressure measured by conventional clinical methods can be treated on the basis of supportive evidence provided by their personal or family history, or by the results of their physical examinations and standard diagnostic tests. It is the patient with persistent but mild hypertension, and in whom there are no other positive findings, who can benefit most from automated blood pressure monitoring.

WHOLE-DAY MONITORING: ESTABLISHING THE TECHNIQUE

The modern ambulatory blood pressure monitors are small portable devices that use noninvasive cuff techniques to obtain repetitive blood pressure measurements throughout a 24-hr period. Typically, these instruments perform their measurements at 15-min intervals. There are two separate methods used by the modern monitoring devices: auscultatory and oscillometric. The ascultatory employs a microphone or transducer positioned beneath the cuff and overlying the brachial artery; it determines systolic and diastolic blood pressures during deflation of the cuff by listening for the Korotkoff sounds. Because these machines can make erroneous readings based on external artifactual sounds, they commonly employ chest leads that provide electrocardiographic R-wave gating for discriminating the true Korotkoff sounds. The oscillometric devices depend upon their perception of fluctuations in the brachial artery itself. This method directly palpates for the systolic blood pressure, and then uses an estimate of the pulse pressure to provide a value for the mean blood pressure. From these measurements, the device then uses an algorithm to calculate the diastolic blood pressure.

Accuracy

Although most ambulatory blood pressure monitoring procedures are performed with noninvasive devices, some investigators have continued to work with portable intra-arterial monitoring equipment. There has been a temptation to use direct intra-arterial measurements as a basis for judging the accuracy of the noninvasive methods. Comparisons of the two methods during 24-hr monitoring periods have shown apparently wide discrepancies between simultaneously obtained intra-arterial and noninvasive measurements (12). Thus, some reservations have been expressed about the validity and accuracy of the noninvasive methods (13). Scrutiny of these data, however, suggests that although patients may exhibit differences between intra-arterial and noninvasive readings, these differences appear to be reasonably consistent throughout the 24-hr period within individual subjects (12).

An assumption underlying this debate has been that the values provided by the intra-arterial measurements represent the true blood pressure. But it could be argued, equally well, that what we know of the natural history and clinical characteristics of hypertension has come from noninvasive cuff measurements. Indeed, except for acute studies, mostly in the in-hospital setting, there is as yet no established basis for interpreting intra-arterial measurements. We have recently used intra-arterial measurements obtained in hospitalized patients as a basis for comparing different noninvasive techniques (14). Figure 1 shows the correlations between blood pressures measured simultaneously by intra-arterial monitoring and by either oscillometric or auscultatory portable devices. Additionally, this figure shows the relationship between intra-arterial values and measurements obtained by the conventional mercury sphygmomanometer. These correlations, although statistically significant, indicate that there are discrepancies between the intra-arterial measurements and those obtained by the various noninvasive methods.

Because the mercury device has long been the standard of measurement, we additionally evaluated the relationships between blood pressures measured by either the oscillometric or auscultatory devices and those provided by the sphygmomanometer. Figure 2 indicates that these correlations are strong, and thus gives confidence that blood pressures provided by the portable devices are a good reflection of sphygmomanometer-based readings. It is important to emphasize that these studies of accuracy have been carried out in

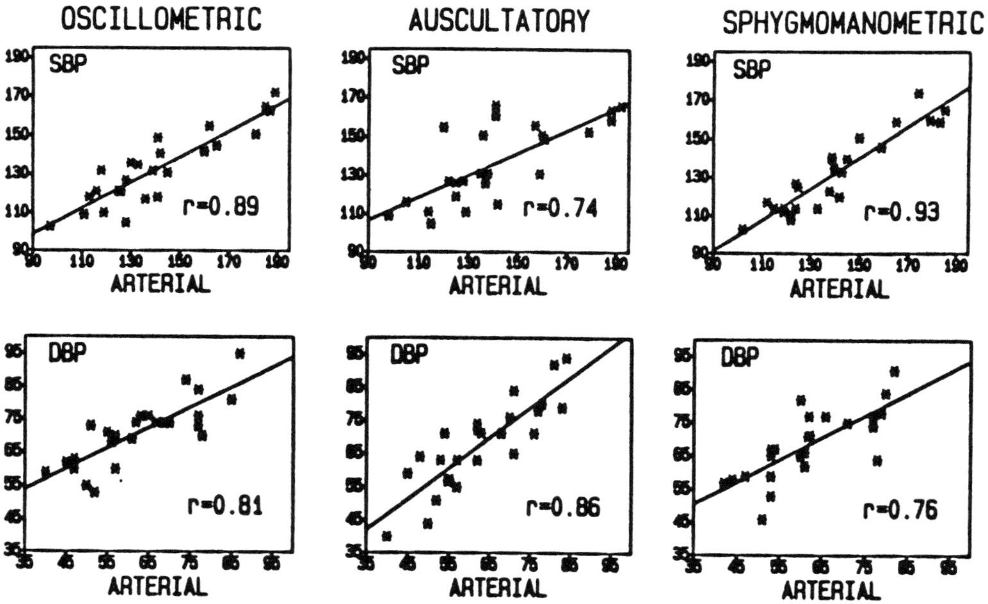

FIG. 1. Relationships between blood pressures measured intra-arterially and by oscillometric or auscultatory portable devices or by a mercury sphygmomanometer in 25 hospitalized patients. Data shown are for systolic blood pressures (SBP) and diastolic blood pressures (DBP). All correlations are significant ($p<.001$ in each case).

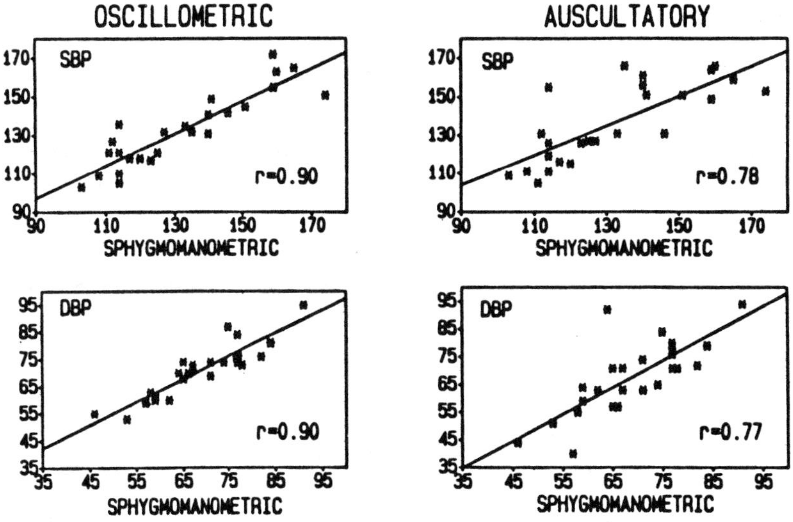

FIG. 2. Relationships between blood pressures measured by a mercury sphygmomanometer and oscillometric or auscultatory devices in 25 hospitalized patients. Data shown are for systolic blood pressures (SBP) and diastolic blood pressures (DBP). All correlations are significant ($p<.001$) in each case).

patients or volunteers in a relatively quiet setting. It has not yet been established whether the portable equipment provides accurate readings during vigorous motion. When instructing patients who are about to undertake the monitoring procedure, it is prudent to advise that they restrict their physical activity.

Physiological Validity

Studies to verify the clinical relevance of the blood pressure monitoring procedure have focused on three characteristics of the whole-day blood pressure: its reproducibility, its ability to describe a circadian pattern, and its relationship to underlying cardiovascular status. The reproducibility of the 24-hr blood pressure has been documented in studies with intra-arterial or noninvasive monitoring (15,16). Of particular interest, the actual circadian pattern of the blood pressure, independently of the blood pressure values themselves, appears to be highly reproducible (16). The 24-hr patterns of blood pressure shown in Fig. 3 were obtained in normal volunteers carrying out their routine daily activities. It is evident that the blood pressure patterns obtained during 24-hr monitoring periods separated by several weeks are superimposable (16).

The characteristic pattern of blood pressure describes a plateau

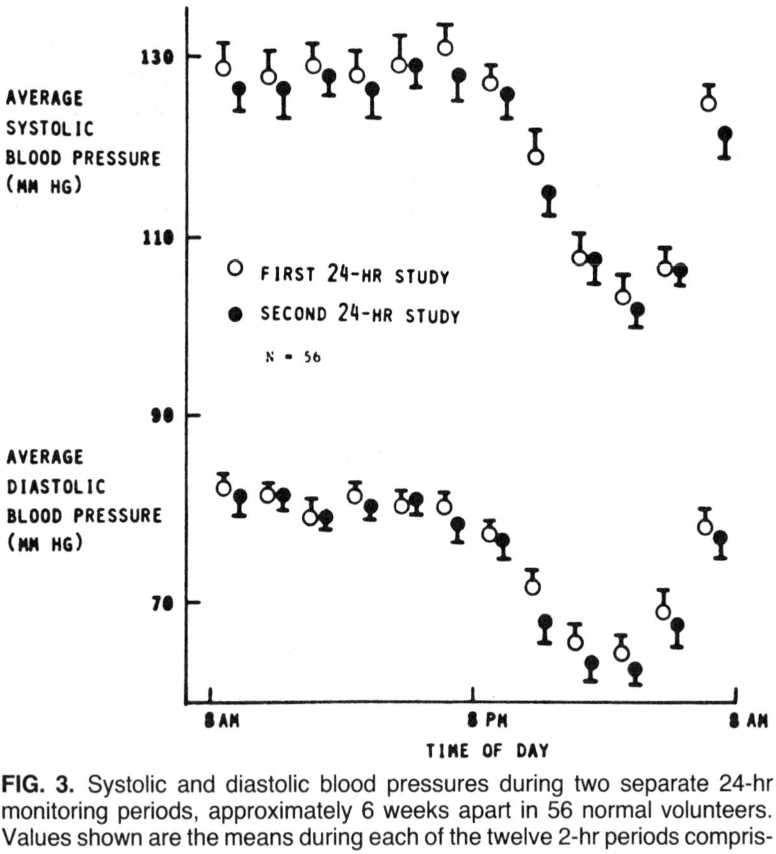

FIG. 3. Systolic and diastolic blood pressures during two separate 24-hr monitoring periods, approximately 6 weeks apart in 56 normal volunteers. Values shown are the means during each of the twelve 2-hr periods comprising the whole day.

during the daytime hours, followed by a decline to nadir values between midnight and 2 AM. Of particular interest is the sharp early morning rise in blood pressure that may originate before awakening and continue through to the early to midmorning hours. It is likely that these morning blood pressure changes reflect the parallel increase in sympathetic nervous system activity that is associated with the arousal process (17). Increasing attention is being paid to the morning pressure peaks, for it has been shown that a relatively large proportion of such major events as myocardial infarctions and strokes occur during this period (18,19). Attention to this time of day can be of value in the diagnostic assessment of patients, and is especially important in evaluating the efficacy of antihypertensive therapy.

A powerful argument favoring the relevance of the whole-day blood pressure is that it correlates more closely than conventional readings with evidence for changes in cardiovascular organs. Investigators have demonstrated, for example, that the values obtained from automated blood pressure monitoring predict echocardiographically measured left ventricular muscle mass far more closely than conventional readings (20,21). Other studies that have employed additional evidence for cardiovascular involvement, including changes in the optic fundi and clinical assessments of the heart in renal function, also have confirmed the clinical relevance of ambulatory blood pressure monitoring.

EXPERIENCE IN NORMALS

The key to the evaluation of the patient with borderline hypertension is to decide whether or not a diagnosis of treatment-requiring hypertension should be made. It would be convenient if simple criteria could be established with ambulatory blood pressure monitoring that would readily allow this important discrimination to be made. However, as we have already discussed, there never has been a clear dividing line, and several factors will determine where in the risk continuum of blood pressure a therapeutic decision should be made in individual patients. Nevertheless, the wise use of automated blood pressure monitoring in such patients would be facilitated by knowledge of blood pressure characteristics in normal controls.

Certain properties of the whole-day blood pressure in normal subjects have already been discussed. It is reproducible and follows a clear circadian pattern. And even within the conventionally accepted normal ranges, the whole-day blood pressure has a relationship to such cardiovascular measurements as echocardiographic left ventricular muscle mass (22).

Effects of Age

Based on conventional blood pressure readings, it has become apparent that blood pressure changes as a function of age. The systolic values tend to increase throughout the life span, whereas the diastolic blood pressure increases less steeply and reaches a plateau in middle age. Thus, there is a progressive widening of the pulse pressure, especially in older individuals. Although we have depended primarily upon diastolic blood pressures for diagnostic criteria, epidemiologic evidence now points to the systolic values as having greater prognostic significance. In studies with whole-day blood pressure monitoring in elderly hypertensive patients, we have found that systolic blood pressure is consistently higher than in younger hypertensive patients, and that diastolic pressures on average are lower (23). It has also been noted that the variability of systolic blood pressure is greater than that for diastolic blood pressure within older patients, and is significantly greater than the variability of systolic blood pressures in younger hypertensive patients. Unfortunately, similar data within a normotensive group of subjects are not available. It is likely that variability of systolic blood pressure in all older people is higher than in younger individuals, but this has not yet been established. Moreover, there has been no agreement concerning the level of continually measured systolic blood pressure that separates normal subjects from those with hypertension, again making it difficult to characterize normalcy of the whole-day blood pressure in older individuals.

It has been shown that whereas approximately two-thirds of elderly hypertensive patients exhibit the usual nocturnal decrease in blood pressure, others maintain their high levels of blood pressure throughout the 24-hr period (24). This may have cardiovascular prognostic significance, for the incidence of complications was higher in the patients who failed to exhibit the nocturnal fall in blood pressure. Whether this differential pattern is a result of ongoing hypertension and its cardiovascular sequelae, or whether such differences in the blood pressure pattern may be of predictive value in normal subjects or those with minimally increased blood pressures, remains to be determined.

A collaborative study has attempted to characterize whole-day patterns of blood pressure in almost 200 normal volunteers subdivided into different age groups (25). A weakness in this study is that it used the same entry criteria (systolic blood pressure less than 140 mmHg) for elderly participants as for the young, thereby making it difficult to evaluate potentially key properties of systolic blood pressure in the elderly. This study noted that the increase in diastolic blood pressures during the hours of work was significantly greater in older than in younger individuals, even though both groups had similar resting blood pressures. There was also a tendency for the variability of blood pressure throughout the day to be greater in the older participants.

The Dividing Line

The choice of a blood pressure level below which values can be regarded as normal inevitably is arbitrary. Because the average of blood pressures obtained throughout the full 24-hr period represented is simple to calculate and is reproducible within individual patients, there has been a tendency to use this value in formulating criteria. The origin of one approach to establishing a dividing line between normal and hypertensive readings is shown in Fig. 4 and is based on observations in groups of normal controls and hypertensive patients. On average, the difference between the whole-day blood pressure averages and carefully measured office readings were 10 mmHg for systolic values and 5 mmHg for diastolic values. Thus, subtracting these differences from 140/90 mmHg, which is the recommended upper limit for normalcy based on conventional

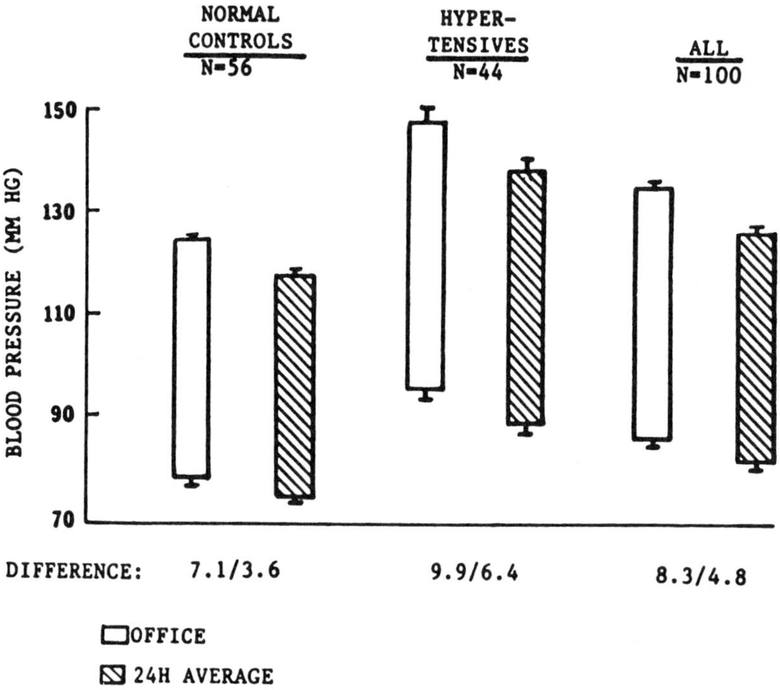

FIG. 4. Mean values for office blood pressures and 24-hr average blood pressures in normal volunteers, hypertensive patients, and all subjects together. The mean systolic and diastolic differences between the office and the 24-hr averages are shown beneath each group.

values (1), gives a whole-day criterion of 130/85 mmHg. Importantly, two other investigators, using differing reasoning (26,27), also have recommended that 130/85 mmHg be the dividing line between normal and hypertensive whole-day blood pressures. From a clinical point of view, most physicians use office readings of 160 mmHg or even higher as their indication for treating isolated or predominant systolic hypertension. It is not yet possible to recommend corresponding whole-day systolic blood pressures for making this diagnosis.

The designation "white-coat" hypertension refers to patients whose whole-day blood pressure values clearly are lower than their office measurements. The same phenomenon also occurs in normal subjects. Figure 5 shows for individual subjects, previously diag-

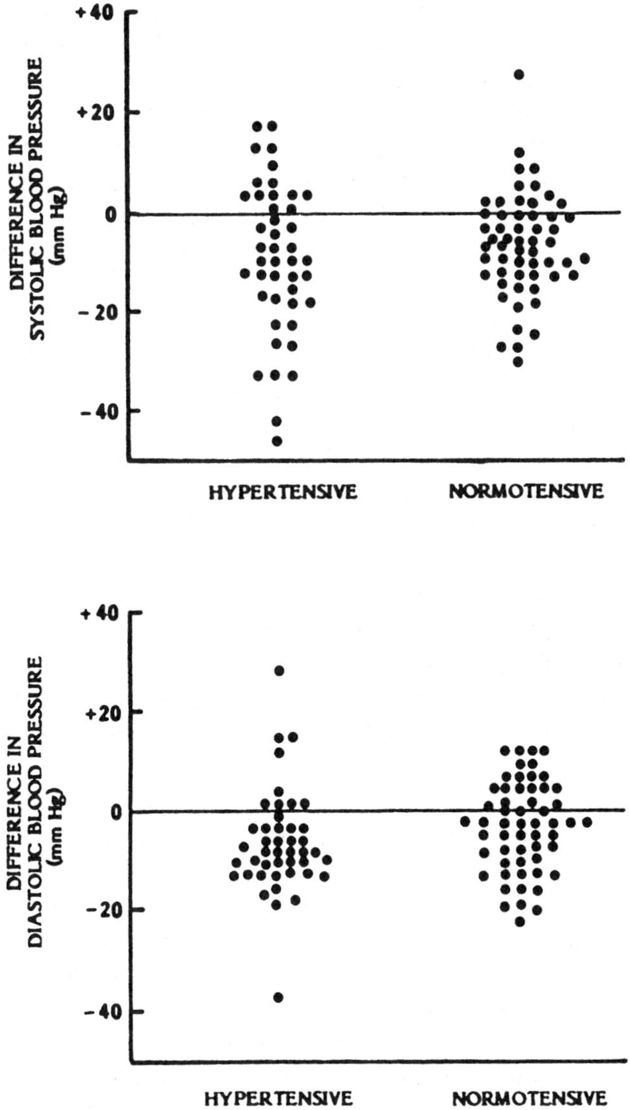

FIG. 5. Differences between office and 24-hr average systolic and diastolic blood pressures shown for individual hypertensive patients and normal volunteers. Values shown below the line indicate 24-hr average was lower than office reading; values shown above the line indicate that the 24-hr average was higher.

nosed by conventional means as having either hypertension or normal blood pressure, the differences between their office readings and their whole-day averages. For both groups there is a tendency for the whole-day averages to be lower than the office readings, presumably reflecting the lower nighttime readings that are incorporated into the whole-day average. It is likely that many of the hypertensive patients whose whole-day averages are substantially lower than their office readings are individuals with "white-coat" hypertension.

It is interesting to note, based on the data shown in Fig. 5, that there are patients in both the hypertensive and normotensive groups whose blood pressures throughout the day actually are higher than their office readings. Thus, the severity of hypertension can be underestimated by standard clinical measurements in some patients. Indeed, it is possible that certain individuals whose office blood pressures fall within the normal range might, in reality, be hypertensive. This false negative aspect of the office blood pressure measurement previously has not been given much consideration. But it may be helpful in patients whose office readings are toward the upper end of the normal range, especially if there is any evidence for other cardiovascular changes or for a revealing family history, to perform whole-day automated blood pressure monitoring.

Application of Monitoring in Borderline Hypertension

Studies with both noninvasive and intra-arterial monitoring devices have demonstrated convincingly that a substantial proportion of patients, especially those with milder forms of hypertension, appear to be hypertensive only when in the presence of physicians or other health personnel. As described elsewhere in this volume, the appearance of a physician produces an alerting reaction in susceptible patients that can increase blood pressures by more than 20 mmHg systolic and 10 mmHg diastolic (7). Serial measurements do not appear to attenuate this phenomenon, although if measurements are repeated after 20 or 30 min there is a tendency for the initial blood pressure response to diminish.

Studies performed in large outpatient hypertensive groups have demonstrated that between 20 and 50% of patients previously diagnosed as having mild to moderate hypertension appear to be normotensive when studied by monitoring throughout the day (26–28). An example of this phenomenon is shown in Fig. 6. This study compared whole-day blood pressure averages in pairs of age-matched hypertensive and normotensive men (28). The diagnosis of hypertension originally had been based on repeated office diastolic blood pressure readings exceeding 90 mmHg, whereas all readings in the normal controls had been below 90 mmHg. Although there is a tendency for the whole-day systolic and diastolic blood pressure averages to be higher in the hypertensive group than in the normal controls, there is clearly some overlap in their values. Approximately one-quarter of the hypertensive men appear to have values that fall within the normal range despite the care with which their earlier office readings had been taken.

An equally strong example of the same problem is shown in Fig. 7. The 15 patients shown in this figure were participants in a rigorously controlled clinical trial of antihypertensive therapy (6). The values for their office diastolic blood pressures shown on the left side of the figure were obtained after several weeks of placebo therapy; indeed several patients had already been excluded from the study because their initially hypertensive readings had fallen below the study's diagnostic criterion during the lengthy lead-in period. Moreover, the office readings had been carefully obtained after patients had been comfortably seated for at least 5 min and represent the averages of duplicate measurements. But, as shown on the right side of Fig. 7, 6 of the 15 patients had normal whole-day blood pressure averages, even though the diagnostic criterion had been appropriately lowered by 5 mmHg (as discussed earlier).

Use in the Clinical Setting

Automated whole-day blood pressure monitoring with automated devices has the capability of discriminating between hypertensive and normotensive individuals whose conventionally measured blood pressures fall into a borderline range. Simpler clinical alternatives to this procedure are less helpful in making this distinction.

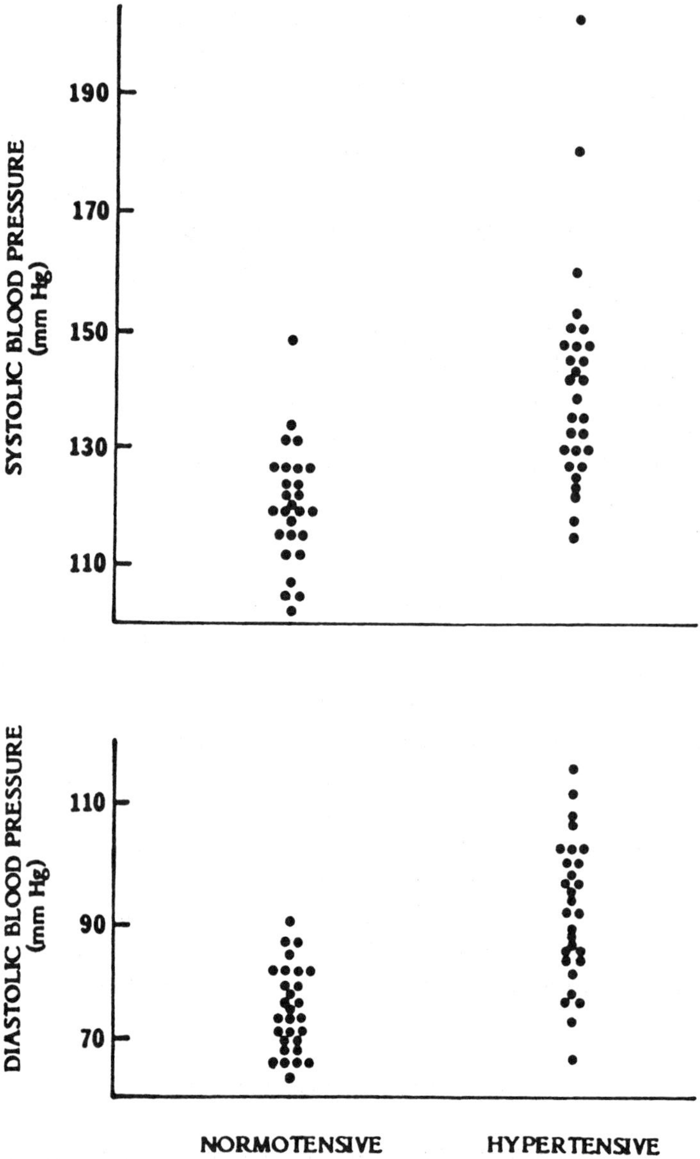

FIG. 6. Whole-day systolic and diastolic blood pressure averages in 29 age-matched pairs of hypertensive and normotensive men.

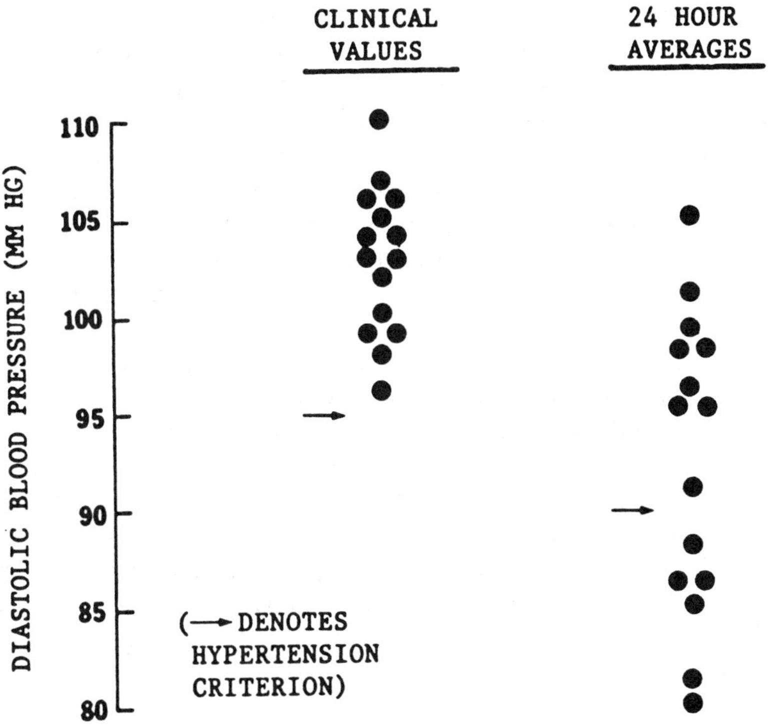

FIG. 7. Conventional clinical diastolic blood pressure measurements and 24-hr diastolic blood pressure averages in 15 hypertensive patients receiving placebo prior to a clinical trial. Values shown above the *arrows* indicate that the criterion for diagnosing hypertension was satisfied.

Despite the greatest possible care in the office measurement of blood pressure, a meaningful number of patients are misdiagnosed. Repeated visits, even over periods of several weeks, cannot guarantee the absence of "white-coat" hypertension. Self-measured blood pressures by the patients, sometimes referred to as "home" blood pressures, also have been advocated as an alternative to the more complex monitoring procedure. Unfortunately, there are no clear criteria for evaluating blood pressures obtained at home or in other settings. The question of time of day is particularly important, for as discussed earlier blood pressure follows a circadian pattern. Typically, blood pressure tends to be relatively low at those hours of the day when patients generally are at home and able to check their blood pressures. Thus, discrepancies between office and home blood pressure measurements simply may reflect the influence of the circadian pattern and potentially could lead to the wrongful exclusion of the diagnosis of hypertension.

Important issues with ambulatory whole-day monitoring still remain to be settled. Perhaps the pivotal question is as follows: Is the patient with office hypertension, but whose whole-day blood pressure values are within the normal range, truly normal? Is the cardiovascular prognosis of such a person identical to that of an individual whose blood pressures are normal in the clinical setting? In an earlier study of young patients with apparently mild hypertension, we found that these individuals had echocardiographic evidence of increased left ventricular muscle wall thickness (29). Although whole-day blood pressure monitoring was not employed in that study, some patients subsequently were found to have normal blood pressures; interestingly, despite their apparent reversion to normotensive status, their echocardiographic measurements of wall thickness were not different from those in patients whose hypertension was sustained. This important question is presently the subject of ongoing prospective research protocols.

SUMMARY

Most patients with hypertension have untreated blood pressures that are only mildly elevated. Thus, small variation in blood pressure measurements can determine whether or not treatment is necessary. The importance of this issue has been shown by major clinical trials in which cardiovascular complications in actively treated patients were only slightly less common than in placebo groups. An explanation for this finding is that placebo patients did better than expected, perhaps due to the dilutional effects of including many participants who eventually were found to be normotensive.

The treatment decision in patients with borderline hypertension can be accomplished in two ways: broad clinical assessment or automated whole-day blood pressure monitoring. Patients with mildly increased conventionally measured blood pressures probably should be treated if they have such concurrent risk factors as lipid abnormalities, diabetes mellitus, or left ventricular hypertrophy; moreover, evidence for early cardiovascular changes, or a family history of hypertension or premature cardiovascular events normally will justify treatment. In patients with mild hypertension, unsupported by other clinical findings, blood pressure monitoring can be very helpful. The newer noninvasive portable devices are accurate and produce whole-day measurements that can demonstrate the circadian blood pressure pattern. The 24-hr measurements are reproducible and are superior to conventional readings as predictors of underlying cardiovascular status. Several investigators have demonstrated that this technique can discriminate normotensive from hypertensive individuals, thereby preventing diagnostic problems of the alerting reaction and office hypertension. Additionally, this diagnostic approach may help identify patients, especially those with early cardiovascular changes or family histories, who are probably hypertensive despite normal or near-normal conventional blood pressure readings.

REFERENCES

1. The 1988 Report of the Joint National Committee on Detection, Evaluation, and Treatment of High Blood Pressure. *Arch Intern Med* 1988;148:1023–1038.
2. Veterans Administration Cooperative Study Group on Antihypertensive Agents. Effects of treatment on morbidity in hypertension. Results in patients with diastolic blood pressures averaging 115 through 129 mmHg. *JAMA* 1967;202:1028–1034.
3. Medical Research Council Working Party. MRC trial of treatment of mild hypertension: principal results. *Br Med J* 1985;291:97–104.
4. Report by the Management Committee. The Australian Therapeutic Trial in Mild Hypertension. *Lancet* 1980;1:1261–1267.
5. Drayer JIM, Weber MA. Monotherapy of essential hypertension with a converting enzyme inhibitor. *Hypertension* 1983;5:180–183.
6. Weber MA, Cheung DG, Graettinger WF, Lipson JL. Characterization of antihypertensive therapy by whole-day BP monitoring. *JAMA* 1988;259:3281–3285.
7. Mancia G, Parati G, Pomidossi G, Grassi G, Casadei R, Zanchetti A. Alerting reaction and rise in blood pressure during measurement by physician and nurse. *Hypertension* 1987;9:209–215.
8. Finnerty FA Jr. Step-down treatment of mild systemic hypertension. *Am J Cardiol* 1984;53:1304–1307.
9. Scannapieco G, Pauletto P, Pagnan A, Mattiello A, Biffanti S, Jori G, Dal

Palu C. Lipoprotein binding to cultured aortic smooth muscle cells from normotensive and hypertensive rats. *J Hypertens* 1988;6(suppl 4):s269–s271.
10. Sammelsson O, Wilmhelmsen L, Anderson OK, Pennert K, Berglund G. Cardiovascular morbidity in relation to change in blood pressure and serum cholesterol levels in treated hypertension. *JAMA* 1987;285:1768–1776.
11. Parving, HH, Anderson AR, Smidt UM, Hommel E, Mathiesen ER, Suendsen PA. Effect of antihypertensive treatment on kidney function in diabetic nephropathy. *Br Med J* 1987;294:1443–1447.
12. Palatini P, Pessina AC, Sperti G, et al. Comparison between an indirect and a direct method of ambulatory blood pressure monitoring. In: Stott FD, Raferty EB, Clement DL, eds. *Proceedings of the 4th International Symposium on Ambulatory Monitoring*. London: Academic Press, 1982;449.
13. Mancia G, Parati G. Experience with 24-hour ambulatory blood pressure monitoring in hypertension. *Am Heart J* 1988;1134–1140.
14. Graettinger WF, Lipson JL, Cheung DG, Weber MA. Validation of portable noninvasive blood pressure monitoring devices: Comparisons with intraarterial and sphygmomanometer measurements. *Am Heart J* 1988;116:1155.
15. Raftery EB. Understanding hypertension: the contribution of direct ambulatory blood pressure monitoring. In: Weber MA. Drayer JIM, eds. *Ambulatory blood pressure monitoring*. Springer-Verlag, 1984;105–116.
16. Weber MA, Drayer JIM, Nakamura DK, Wyle FA. The circadian blood pressure pattern in ambulatory normal subjects. *Am J Cardiol* 1984;54:115–119.
17. Linsell CR, Lightman SL, Mullen PE, Brown MJ, Causon RC. Circadian rhythms of epinephrine and norepinephrine in man. *J Clin Endocrinol Metab* 1985;60:1210–1215.
18. Agnoli A, Manfredi M, Mossuto L, Piccinelli A. Rapport entre les rythmes hemeronyctaux de la tensionarterielle et sa pathogenie de l'insuffisance vasculaire cerebrale. *Rev Neurol* 1975;131:597–606.
19. Meyers A, Dewar HA. Circumstances attending 100 sudden deaths from coronary artery disease with coroners' necropsies. *Br Heart J* 1975;37:1133–1143.
20. Drayer JIM, Weber MA, DeYoung JL. BP as a determinant of cardiac left ventricular muscle mass. *Arch Intern Med* 1983;143:90–92.
21. Devereux RB, Pickering TG, Harshfield GA, et al. Left ventricular hypertrophy in patients with hypertension: importance of blood pressure response to regularly recurring stress. *Circulation* 1983;68:470–476.
22. Drayer JIM, Gardin JM, Brewer DD, Weber MA. Disparate relationships between blood pressure and left ventricular mass in patients with and without left ventricular hypertrophy. *Hypertension* 1987;6(suppl II):II61–II64.
23. Waeber B, Jacot des Combes B, Porchet M, Brunner AR. Accuracy, reproducibility and usefulness of ambulatory blood pressure recording obtained with the Remler system. In: Weber MA, Drayer JIM, eds. *Ambulatory blood pressure monitoring*. Steinkopff, Darmstadt, 1984;65–69.
24. Weber MA, Drayer JIM, Nakamura DK, Wyle FA. The circadian blood pressure pattern in ambulatory normal subjects. *Am J Cardiol* 1984;54:115–119.
25. Weber MA, Drayer JIM, Chard ER. Blood pressure fluctuation and amplitude in normal human subjects. In: Weber MA, Drayer JIM, eds. Ambulatory blood pressure monitoring. Springer-Verlag, 1984;43–50.
26. Pickering TG, James GD, Boddie C, Harshfield GA, Blank S, Laragh JH. How common is white coat hypertension? *JAMA* 1988;259:225–228.

27. Krakoff, LR, Eison H, Phillips RH, Leiman SJ, Lev S. Effect of ambulatory blood pressure monitoring on the diagnosis and cost of treatment for mild hypertension. *Am Heart J* 1988;116:1152.
28. Drayer JIM, Weber MA, Nakamura DK. Automated ambulatory blood pressure monitoring: a study in age-matched normotensive and hypertensive men. *Am Heart J* 1985;109:1334–1338.
29. Weber MA, Drayer JIM, Baird WM. Echocardiographic evaluation of left ventricular hypertrophy. *J Cardiovasc Pharmacol* 1986;8(3):s61–s69.

Ambulatory Blood Pressure Recording,
edited by H. Brunner and B. Waeber.
Raven Press, Ltd., New York © 1992.

6

Home Monitoring of Blood Pressure: An Alternative to Ambulatory Monitoring?

Thomas G. Pickering

Cardiovascular Center, The New York Hospital-Cornell University Medical Center, New York, New York 10021

The realization that blood pressure readings taken by a physician in his office may not be a very reliable guide to the level of blood pressure occurring at other times is not new. Nearly 50 years ago Ayman and Goldshine described their experience with 34 hypertensive patients who had been trained to take their blood pressure at home or have it measured by a family member (1). Almost without exception, the patients recorded lower pressures than the physicians got in their office, in some cases by as much as 70/36 mmHg. Such differences persisted over a 6-month period of observation. The authors suggested that measurement of blood pressure by the patient might have three advantages over the conventional clinic measurements: (a) a better understanding of the factors that influence blood pressure, (b) an improved prediction of prognosis, and (c) a better way of evaluating treatment. Their observations received little attention at the time but have major implications, the most important of which is that some patients may be misclassified as being hypertensive on the basis of their clinic readings, if their pressures are normal outside the clinic. Although clinic pressures still remain the gold standard for defining hypertension for most physicians, there is increasing acceptance that this standard is flawed, and that pressures measured outside the clinic, either at home or by ambulatory monitoring, may help to improve the reliability of the diagnosis in the individual patient. This chapter reviews the uses of home monitoring of blood pressure, and compares it with ambulatory monitoring.

RATIONALE FOR THE USE OF HOME MONITORING: THE UNRELIABILITY OF CLINIC PRESSURES

There are in principle two reasons for recommending the wider use of home blood pressure measurement: (a) the unreliability of clinic pressures, and (b) the greater cost-effectiveness of home monitoring.

There can be little doubt that the presence of the physician has a major influence on the blood pressure recorded during a clinic visit, and is probably the chief explanation for the higher readings obtained in this setting. This was most forcefully demonstrated in two studies conducted by Mancia's group. Using continuous intra-arterial recording of blood pressure in hospitalized patients, they showed that when a physician came up to take a blood pressure reading with a mercury sphygmomanometer on the patient's other arm, there was a marked rise of intra-arterial pressure that persisted throughout the measurement procedure and then gradually subsided (2). Repeated visits by the same physician did not result in any habituation of the response. In a second study, the average rise of pressure evoked by the presence of a physician was 23/18 mmHg, which was approximately twice the rise occuring when a nurse took the blood pressure reading (3). We have also observed that blood pressures measured by a physician tend to be higher than those measured by a technician, and also that the technician's readings are closer to the average daytime level than the physician's (4).

We compared pressures measured in the clinic by the physician with self-measured home pressures in 93 patients with mild untreated hypertension, using the average 24-hr blood pressure measured by an ambulatory monitor as the reference value (5). For both systolic and diastolic pressure the home pressures gave closer correlations than clinic pressures with the average 24-hr pressures (Fig. 1).

One of the reasons why home readings are theoretically more reliable than clinic readings is that a larger number of measurements can be used to characterize an individual's blood pressure. If patients are classified as being hypertensive on the basis of a single clinic visit, a significant overestimate of the prevalence of hypertension is likely to occur. In the Charlottesville blood pressure survey, 20% of adults were classified as hypertensive on initial screening,

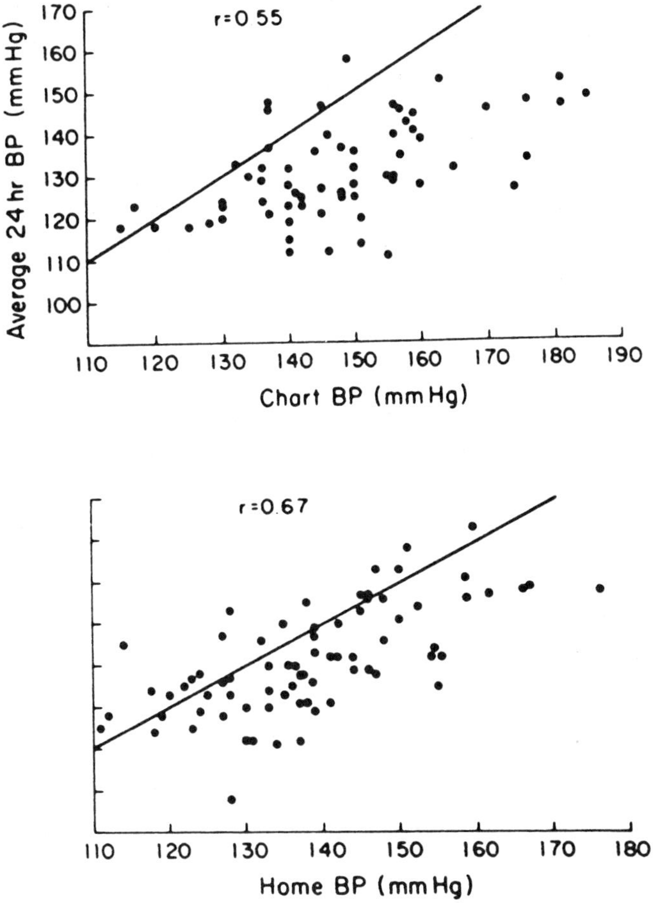

FIG. 1. Comparison of systolic blood pressures measured in the clinic by a physician (*top panel*) and at home by the patient (*bottom panel*) with 24-hr pressures measured by ambulatory monitoring (From ref. 5, with permission).

but this figure fell to 9% with repeated measurements (6). Watson et al. (7) made repeated measurements during 12 clinic visits in a series of hypertensive patients. During the first three visits there was a progressive fall of pressure, but on subsequent visits there was no further systematic change. Because of the significant degree of spontaneous variability of blood pressure between visits, however, they estimated that six visits would be needed to define an individual patient's average level of clinic pressure. Similar trends have been noted in the Framingham study (8), and in the large clinical trials of the treatment of mild hypertension (9,10).

This decline of blood pressure with repeated measurement occurs not only between visits, but also within visits. In a study in which six consecutive readings were taken in one session, systolic pressure fell by 10 mmHg between the first and last readings (over an interval of 25 min), whereas diastolic pressure changed little (11). The fall of systolic pressure was not a function of the patient's age or sex. In another study systolic pressure decreased after four readings by 4 mmHg, and diastolic by 2 mmHg (12). Such changes depend to a large extent on the interval between successive readings: if this is very short no significant falls of pressure may be recorded (13).

In a study of 292 patients with borderline hypertension (defined as a clinic diastolic pressure between 90 and 104 mmHg) we attempted to determine how many such patients had elevations of pressure only in the clinic situation, which we and others have termed "white-coat" hypertension (14). To do this, we compared their 24-hr ambulatory pressures with 24-hr pressures obtained in normotensive individuals. Approximately 20% of the hypertensives had normal ambulatory pressures, suggesting that the exclusive reliance on clinic measurement of blood pressure may lead to a substantial misclassification of patients with hypertension (Fig. 2). Somewhat similar results were obtained by Waeber et al. (15), who performed ambulatory recordings in 245 untreated patients judged to be hypertensive on the basis of their clinic readings (at least 140/90 mmHg). Only 39% had average daytime systolic pressures above 140 mmHg, and 44% diastolics above 90 mmHg.

The traditional argument used in defense of clinic pressures is that they represent the patient's response to the stresses of everyday life, but we were unable to verify this in our study (4). Patients with "white-coat" hypertension did not show any greater variability of blood pressure during ambulatory monitoring, nor did their response to stress, as measured by the difference between home and work blood pressures, appear to be any different. An extreme example of this phenomenon is shown in Fig. 3. This patient, a 64-year-

FIG. 2. Distribution of ambulatory diastolic blood pressure levels in patients with clinic (chart) pressures between 90 and 104 mmHg.

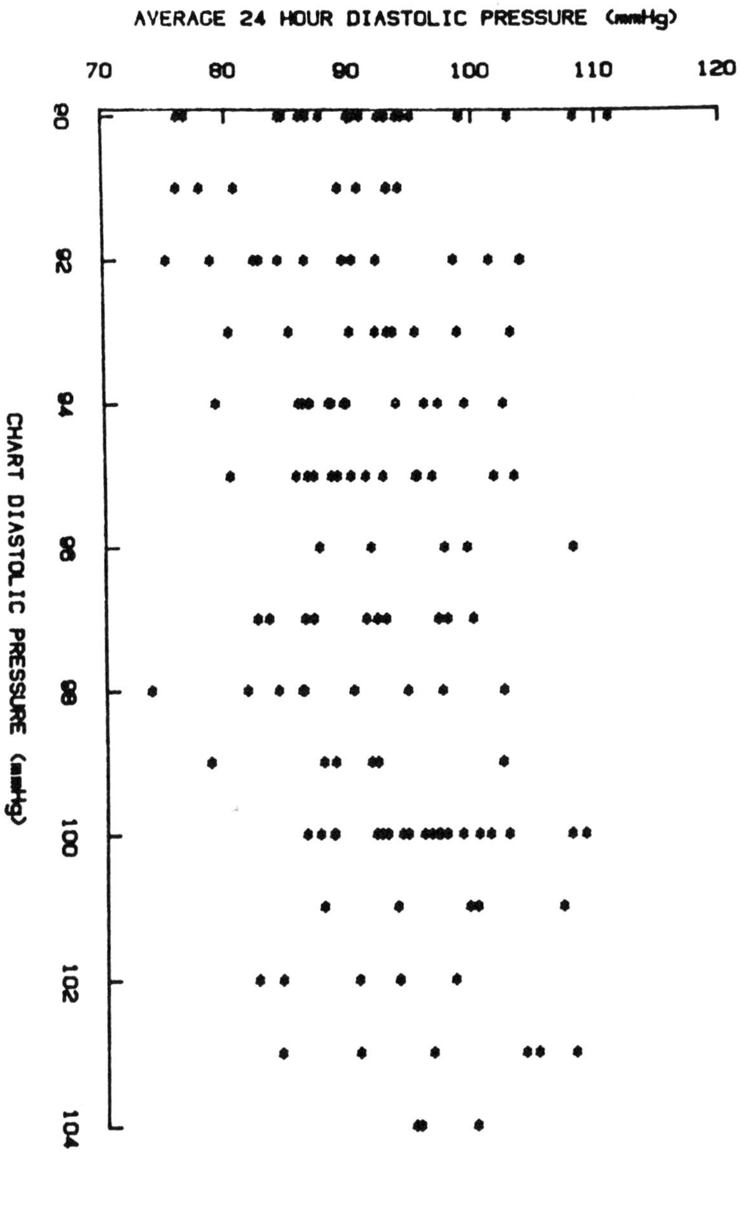
AVERAGE 24 HOUR DIASTOLIC PRESSURE (mmHg)
70
80
90
100
110
120
90
92
94
96
98
100
102
104
CHART DIASTOLIC PRESSURE (mmHg)

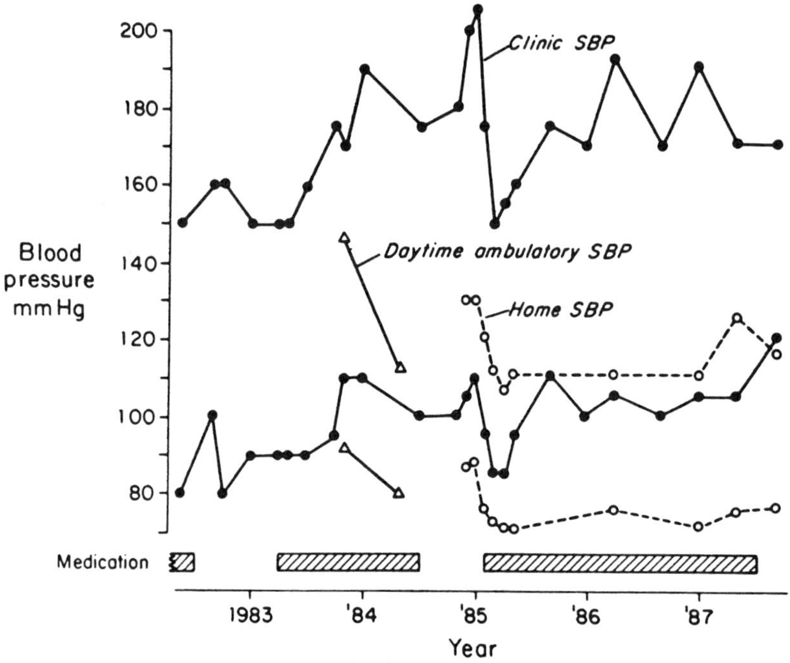

FIG. 3. "White-coat" hypertension in a 64-year-old female, showing clinic, home, and ambulatory systolic and diastolic pressures recorded over a period of several years. (Reproduced from ref. 14, with permission.)

old woman, had persistently elevated clinic pressures for several years, often reaching 180/120 mmHg. Her home pressures, in contrast, have been as low as 120/80 mmHg. That her technique of self-monitoring was accurate was demonstrated by having her take her own pressure in the clinic with her own machine, when she also recorded very high readings. Her ambulatory blood pressures were closer to the home than to the clinic pressures, and echocardiography revealed no evidence of target organ damage.

COMPARISON OF HOME AND CLINIC PRESSURES

The original observation of Ayman and Goldshine that home pressures are usually much lower than clinic pressures has been confirmed in a number of studies. In patients with severe hypertension Corcoran et al. (16) reported that clinic pressures were on average

20/10 mmHg higher than home readings, and that these clinic readings were also higher than readings taken in hospital by a nurse (16). In mildly hypertensive subjects Laughlin et al. (17) found clinic pressures to be 11/5 mmHg higher than home pressure, and in our own study there was a similar difference of 10/5 mmHg (5). Badskjaer and Nielsen (18) reported an average difference of 13/3 mmHg, but there was no correlation between the home and clinic pressure. Laughlin et al. (19) reported in a second study that home pressures showed a progressive decline with repeated measurement, which we did not find; in our subjects the average pressures measured during the 1st and 3rd week of home recordings were the same. Kenny et al. (20) measured blood pressure by four different techniques on three occasions separated by intervals of 2 weeks in 19 patients with borderline hypertension. The techniques included conventional clinic measurement, basal blood pressure (measured after lying for 30 min in a quiet room), daytime ambulatory pressure, and self-recorded home pressure. None of the four measures showed any consistent change over the 3 study days, although there was an insignificant downward trend in all of them. For all 3 days, the clinic pressures were consistently higher than any of the other measures, but there were no significant differences between any of the other three measures. The average difference between clinic and home pressures was 9/4 mmHg.

In another study comparing the reproducibility of home, clinic, and ambulatory pressures we took two sets of each type of measurement separated by an interval of 2 weeks (21). In hypertensive patients we found a significant decline of systolic pressure in the clinic over this period, but the home and ambulatory pressures showed no significant change (Fig. 4). In normotensive subjects there was no consistent change in any of the three measures of blood pressure. These findings support the notion that the fall of clinic pressure is largely spurious, and primarily due to habituation to the clinic setting.

In normotensive subjects the differences between clinic and home pressures are much smaller (15). In an epidemiological population survey Welin et al. (22) found only minor differences. These investigators also reported that subjects who were most familiar with the clinic setting exhibited the smallest differences between the home and clinic readings. Similar results were reported by Beckman et al.

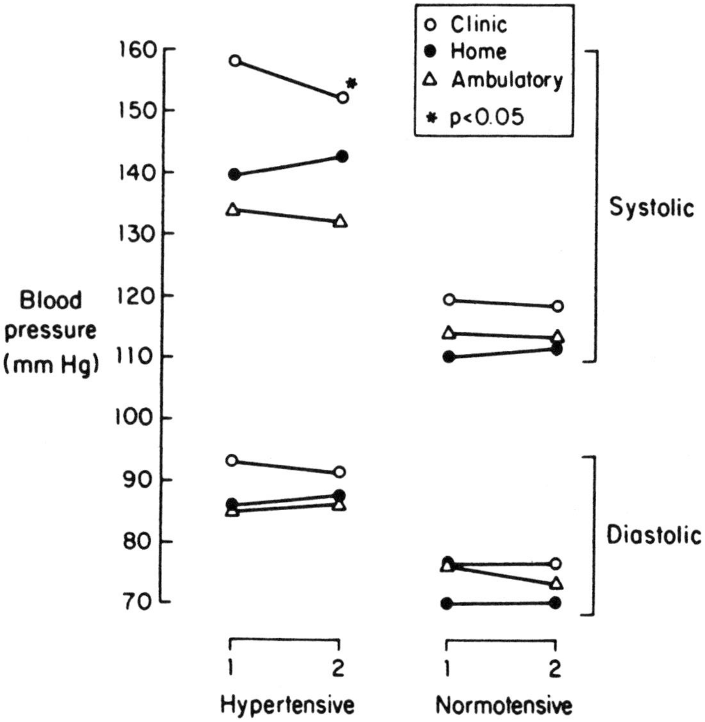

FIG. 4. Comparison of home, clinic, and ambulatory pressures measured on two occasions 2 weeks apart.

(23), who found that subjects labeled as being mildly hypertensive had systolic pressures 15 mmHg higher in the clinic than at home, whereas in normotensives this difference was only 2 mmHg. Finally, Julius et al. (24) reported a mean difference of 14/4 mmHg between clinic and home readings in a series of patients with borderline hypertension, but no difference (1/ − 3 mmHg) in normotensives.

The fact that numerous studies have found that the differences between clinic and home pressures is greater in patients with borderline hypertension than in normotensive subjects raises an interesting paradox. Since hypertension is conventionally defined by the level of pressure measured in the clinic rather than at home, individuals who happen to show an exaggerated blood pressure response to the clinic setting will be selected out and labeled as hypertensive. The reason why the clinic setting raises blood pressure more in some individuals than in others hence assumes considerable importance. The anxiety associated with a clinic visit is the most obvious explanation, but we believe that it is not the whole story. Two studies have failed to show any correlation between the clinic-home difference and psychometric evaluations of state and trait anxiety (17,25). We have suggested elsewhere (15,26) that one of the initiating factors may be the patient's perception of the physician as a potentially threatening authority figure, which results in the increased clinic pressure. With many subjects this response habituates with repeated exposure, leading to their classification as normotensive individuals. With others, however, this habituation does not occur, and these individuals are labeled as hypertensive. One way by which this could take place is that when the patient is told at the first visit that the pressure is high, and needs to be rechecked on a subsequent visit, the pressor response is once more elicited, and becomes self-perpetuating as part of a classically conditioned response to the stimulus of the physician and the clinic. Some experimental support for this mechanism was provided by a recent study (27) in which 29 young men who were found to have elevated blood pressure on a routine examination were divided into two groups. The first was sent a letter telling them that their pressure was too high, and the second a neutral letter. On the second examination the blood pressure in the first group was 16/10 mmHg higher than in the second group throughout a 45-min testing period. This study demonstrates that the patient's expectation may have a profound effect on the blood pressure.

FACTORS INFLUENCING HOME BLOOD PRESSURE LEVELS

As with any other measure of blood pressure, the level of pressure that is recorded during home monitoring shows considerable variability, and is likely to be influenced by a number of factors.

The one that has received most attention is the time of day. In most westernized societies a large proportion of people are at work during the middle of the day, so that the only practical time for recording home blood pressures is before going to work in the morning, or after they get home in the evening. In three studies where morning and evening measurements were both taken, the evening readings tended to be higher for systolic pressure (by about 3 mmHg), but there were no consistent differences for diastolic pressure (19,22,28). When the pressures are recorded in the afternoon, they are likely to be the highest of the day (23,28).

There is relatively little information as to whether pressures recorded on non-workdays are the same as on workdays. Welin et al. (22) concluded that there were no differences, but in a study using ambulatory monitoring of blood pressure we found that the pressure at home in the evening was consistently higher if the patient had gone to work earlier in the day (29).

Diastolic blood pressure tends to fall after a meal, but the change is usually relatively small (around 3 to 5 mmHg), and systolic pressure is not affected (30). If the patient has recently smoked a cigarette, or drunk coffee, higher readings will be recorded (31). Conversely, if the readings are taken soon after a period of heavy exercise, they are likely to be lower.

TECHNIQUE OF HOME BLOOD PRESSURE MONITORING

Patients can be taught to record home blood pressures with reasonable accuracy. Gould et al. (32) compared self-recorded blood pressures taken with an aneroid sphygmomanometer with simultaneously determined intra-arterial pressures taken with an ambulatory monitor. There was no consistent difference for systolic pressure measured by the two techniques, and only 3 mmHg for diastolic pressure. There was also a reasonably good correlation between the self-monitored and intra-arterial pressure. Furthermore, the average home readings for systolic pressure were in good agreement with the average daytime ambulatory pressures, although home-measured diastolic pressures were less reliable.

The act of inflating one's own sphygmomanometer cuff produces a transient elevation of blood pressure of around 12 mmHg, which lasts only about 10 sec, so that by the time the cuff is deflated to systolic pressure, the pressure has returned to baseline (33). This increase of blood pressure is due to the muscular activity involved in cuff inflation rather than to the compressing effects of the cuff on the arm. If the cuff is deflated too quickly it is possible that the pressure will not have returned to baseline, so that spuriously high systolic pressures may be recorded (34). Patients should therefore be instructed to inflate the cuff more than 30 mmHg above the expected systolic pressure, and to deflate the cuff slowly.

A large number of devices for home monitoring is now available. Virtually all use a sphygmomanometer cuff placed on the upper arm, although there is now at least one which uses a finger cuff. Two general categories are available: automatic and nonautomatic devices. The latter require an observer to listen for the Korotkoff sounds with a stethoscope, whereas the former use some automatic detection mode. The most reliable technique is the traditional mercury sphygmomanometer. It is more expensive than the other nonautomatic device, the aneroid sphygmomanometer, but is also more accurate. Aneroid recorders are satisfactory for most purposes, provided the dials are checked for accuracy against a mercury column. Patients who are using these recorders require training in their proper use.

The automatic devices are rapidly gaining in popularity. They are more expensive than aneroid recorders, but are potentially simpler to use, and eliminate observer bias. We evaluated 11 such devices currently available in the United States, comparing them against simultaneously determined readings taken from the opposite arm by a trained observer using a mercury sphygmomanometer (35). The ideal method of testing would be to connect a mercury column via a T-piece to the cuff of the machine, and have the observer listen for Korotkoff sounds just distal to the blood pressure cuff, which would enable the observer and the machine to take readings simultaneously from the same arm. We did not do this in our survey, however, because with some of the recorders it is not possible to insert a T-piece. When the opposite arm is used, allowance has to be made for the fact that the pressure may not be identical in the two arms, and that the readings will not be simultaneous. We evaluated these factors, and found that about 70% of readings taken in this way will be within 5 mmHg of each other. In our study, only 4 of 11 machines tested gave readings that were consistently within 5 mmHg of the observer's readings (Fig. 5). Differences between machine and observer readings were greatest in patients with higher pressures, when most machines underestimated systolic pressure—by as much as 15 mmHg in one case. Other findings were that systolic pressure was generally more accurately detected than diastolic, and that there was no correlation between the price of the machines and their accuracy.

Other studies have been published on the testing of equipment available in Denmark (36) and Switzerland (37), and have obtained generally similar results: in the Danish study the average deviation of six electronic recorders from auscultatory readings ranged from 1/0 to 13/6 mmHg. One of the problems in comparing these reports is that the same machines, which are mostly of Japanese origin, may be marketed in different countries under different names.

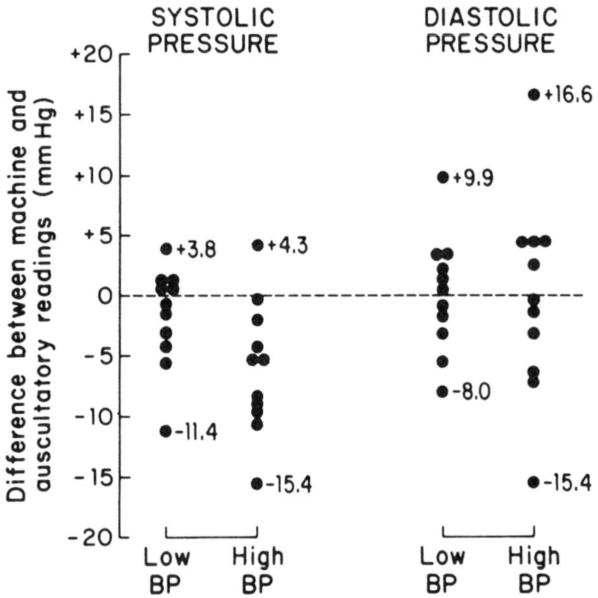

FIG. 5. Comparison of blood pressures measured with a mercury sphygmomanometer and 11 electronic recorders in two groups of subjects (low and high BP).

At the present time there is no enforcement of standards of accuracy for such recorders, either in the United States or Europe, although professional bodies have recommended that this should be undertaken (38,39).

HOME MONITORING FOR THE DIAGNOSIS OF HYPERTENSION

In the initial evaluation of the hypertensive patient, the diagnostic process is mainly concerned with quantifying the elevation of blood pressure, and hence the need for treatment. By providing a convenient and cheap method for increasing the number of readings, home monitoring can greatly reduce the error that is inevitable if only a few clinic readings are used. It has been shown on theoretical grounds that a better estimate of an individual's "true" level of blood pressure can be obtained by taking a few readings each time on several different occasions rather than by taking a larger number on a single occasion (40). It is our custom to ask patients to take readings both in the morning and evening 2 or 3 days a week for at least 3 weeks. This procedure allows time for the patient to become familiar with the measurement procedure, so that a reasonably stable level of pressure can be recorded, and the effects of diurnal variation allowed for.

A potential concern with the use of self-monitoring of blood pressure is that it will increase the patient's anxiety about his or her condition. In practice this has been found usually not to be the case. In one study 70% of patients reported that they found the technique to be reassuring (40).

As discussed above, clinic pressures tend to decrease with repeated visits. In a recent study by Padfield et al. (42) clinic blood pressure was measured on three occasions over a period of 4 weeks. At the first visit the patients were instructed in the use of home monitors, and asked to measure their pressure over 3 days. The pressure at the first clinic visit was higher than the home pressures, but there was no consistent difference between the final clinic pressure and the home pressure. These authors concluded that home blood pressures can be used to predict the results of repeated clinic measurements, and hence may be of use in making therapeutic decisions.

In the first step, if there is evidence from the clinical examination or laboratory tests of target organ damage attributable to the blood pressure, treatment can be started without any further evaluation of the severity of hypertension. If target organ damage is not detected, however, home monitoring is appropriate. If this reveals high readings, e.g., 140/90 mmHg or more, treatment may again be appropriate. If the pressures are less than this, however, an ambulatory recording will resolve whether the clinic or the home pressures are closer to the "true" pressure.

HOME MONITORING FOR THE EVALUATION OF ANTIHYPERTENSIVE TREATMENT

When patients are having their antihypertensive medication initiated or changed it is necessary to measure their blood pressure on repeated occasions. Home monitoring is again ideal for this purpose, because it can obviate the need for many clinic visits. It has the additional advantage of avoiding the biases inherent in clinic pressure measurements.

The greater statistical power inherent in the use of home recordings rather than clinic recordings for the evaluation of antihypertensive medications was well illustrated in a study by Menard et al. (43). They used a double blind, within-patient crossover study, with 2-week periods of three different treatments (a diuretic, a beta blocker, and both together) separated by 2-week placebo periods. They measured blood pressure in the clinic at the end of each treatment period, and patients also recorded their blood pressures at home using a semiautomatic machine. The effectiveness of all three treatment modes was similar for both measures of blood pressure. The greater number of home readings increased the sensitivity of the study to detect a difference of blood pressure between the different treatment modalities. It was estimated that in order to detect a treatment effect of 5 mmHg, 27 patients would be needed if clinic blood pressures were used for the evaluation, but only 20 patients if home pressures were used.

The validity of using home readings for monitoring the effects of treatment on blood pressure is well established. Cottier et al. (44) used small doses of clonidine and propranolol interspersed with blinded placebo periods, and found that home pressures were consistently lower during the periods of active treatment. Gould et al. (45) compared clinic, ambulatory (intra-arterial), and home pressures in two trials, one using verapamil, and other prazosin. For both agents, clinic pressures showed a bigger change than home or ambulatory pressures as a result of treatment, but there was no placebo phase, so that the bigger fall of clinic pressure may have been partly from a placebo response. The changes recorded by intra-arterial monitoring and by home monitoring were generally similar. In a study of 50 patients whose response to antihypertensive medication was monitored both at home and in the clinic, Ibrahim et al. (46) found that when there was a discrepancy between the two measures of blood pressure, electrocardiographic changes of left ventricular hypertrophy correlated most closely with the home pressure.

Home monitoring can also be used for assessing the duration of action of antihypertensive medications. In a study comparing meclothiazide and furosemide, blood pressures were measured both in the clinic and three times a day at home (47). Meclothiazide lowered the pressure throughout the day, whereas the effects of furosemide appeared to be wearing off by the evening.

HOME MONITORING AND COMPLIANCE WITH TREATMENT

Noncompliance with treatment prescribed for hypertension can be a significant barrier to its effective control. One potential way in which this can be overcome is by increasing the involvement of the patient in the treatment process. Home monitoring of blood pressure can help to achieve this. In a study of medication compliance with antihypertensive treatment in Canadian steelworkers, Haynes et al. (48) studied 38 patients whose compliance was poor and whose blood pressure was uncontrolled. These patients were allocated to an experimental or control group. The former patients were instructed in the use of home blood pressure monitoring and pill counting, whereas the latter continued to be evaluated in the clinic in the conventional way. Over a 6-month period this procedure resulted in an improved compliance with medication of 20% and a fall of diastolic pressure of 5 mmHg in the experimental group, but no significant changes in the control group.

COST-EFFECTIVENESS OF HOME MONITORING

It is not hard to make a case for the cost-effectiveness of home blood pressure monitoring. The equipment can be purchased for about $50 for an aneroid sphygmomanometer, or $150 for an automatic monitor. The only other cost involved is in the training of the patient in its proper use, which can be done by a nurse in about half an hour.

The costs saved are considerable. The finding of a normal home blood pressure in a patient with elevated clinic pressures may be an indication that no antihypertensive medication needs to be prescribed, particularly if the ambulatory pressure is also normal. For patients who are starting treatment the number of clinic visits can be curtailed, since it is often possible to adjust the dose of medication over the telephone. For each clinic visit, the cost saved includes not only the fee for the visit, but also the time off work and costs of transportation.

In a recent survey 50 general practitioners in South Wales were asked what interval between clinic visits they would recommend to their hypertensive patients. The average was 15 weeks, but 24% said they would see patients every 2 to 8 weeks (49). Other surveys have reported average follow-up intervals ranging from 1 to 4 months (50,51). It is likely that in many cases, these intervals could be lengthened with greater use of home monitoring.

CAN HOME MONITORING SUBSTITUTE FOR AMBULATORY MONITORING?

Although it is becoming increasingly accepted that clinic readings may be inadequate when used on their own, there is dispute as to whether the extra cost and inconvenience of ambulatory blood pressure monitoring can be justified. Home monitoring is often proposed as an alternative, on the grounds that it is much cheaper and simpler. For the initial evaluation, the most important thing to ascertain is whether the patient is at sufficiently high risk of cardiovascular morbidity as a result of the hypertension to warrant treatment. A large body of data is available to answer this question, but it is almost all based on clinic measurements. Although these give a good estimate of risk for the population as a whole, for the individual patient the prediction is relatively weak. In principle, this prediction could be improved by using additional measures of pressure taken outside the clinic setting, such as home or ambulatory readings. There is unfortunately at the present time little prospective data to answer this important question. Only one large scale prospective study has so far been published, by Perloff et al. (52), which did find that ambulatory pressures improved the prediction of prognosis over what could be predicted from clinic pressures alone. A number of other studies, which we have recently reviewed (53), have demonstrated that ambulatory pressures correlate more closely than clinic pressures with several different indices of target organ damage.

There is even less information on this question for home pressures. No studies have compared the prognostic values of home versus clinic pressures and very few have related home pressures to the severity of target organ damage. Two that did found that echocardiographically determined left ventricular mass correlated more closely with home than with clinic pressures (5,53), as shown in Table 1. It should also be pointed out that many of the blood pressure readings recorded during the ambulatory monitoring studies cited above were taken while the patient was at home. In our own study, however, we found that the correlation between ambulatory blood pressure and left ventricular hypertrophy was closer if the patient went to work during the day of recording than if he or she stayed at home (55).

The other problem with home pressures is that they usually represent the level of pressure at the lower end of the waking range, when the patient is relatively relaxed. Thus, they do not necessarily provide a good guide to what happens to the patient's pressure when

TABLE 1. *Correlations between left ventricular mass and blood pressure measured either at home by self-monitoring or in the clinic*

Reference	*n*	Clinic SBP	Clinic DBP	Home SBP	Home DBP
Kleinert (5)	45	0.22	0.07	0.45	0.40
Verdecchia (54)	34	0.30	—	0.41	—

undergoing the stresses of daily life, such as occur during work. As shown in Fig. 6, the pressure at work tends to be higher than the pressure at home, and closer to the clinic pressure, although the clinic pressure is not necessarily a good guide to the level of pressure at work. In patients with mild hypertension we found only a moderate correlation between home and work blood pressures (r = .55 for systolic, .65 for diastolic pressure) (5). Although the majority of subjects do show a higher pressure at work than at home (56), we have encountered others whose pressure is not lower, or is even higher, at home. This is particularly true of women with children (57).

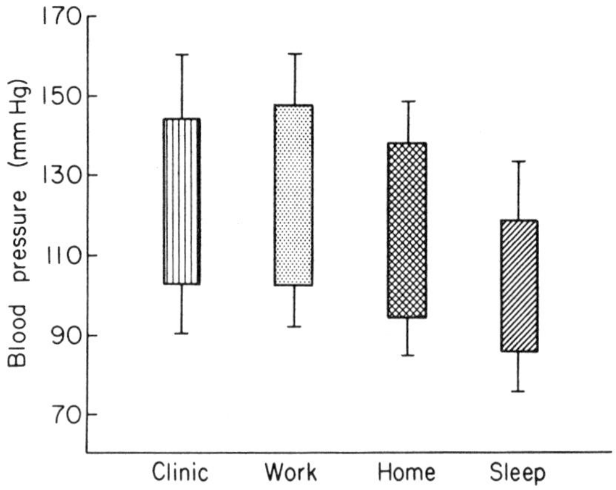

FIG. 6. Comparison of average systolic and diastolic pressures (upper and lower end of bars) in different situations in patients with borderline hypertension.

CONCLUSIONS

The days when physicians could rely solely on clinic measurements of blood pressure for the assessment of patients with known or suspected hypertension are passing. This applies most strongly to patients with mild hypertension, who comprise the majority of the hypertensive population, and in whom relatively small differences in the pressure that is recorded can determine whether or not medication is prescribed. Blood pressure is not a fixed entity, and hence can be more reliably characterized by increasing the number of readings. In addition, the circumstances in which the pressure is measured may have a major effect. The most notable of these is the setting of the clinic or physician's office, which in patients with mild hypertension may raise the systolic pressure by 10 mmHg or more, and the diastolic by about 5 mmHg. It is therefore essential to obtain additional readings of pressure away from the clinic, because many such patients will be normotensive except when they are in the clinic. For this purpose, both home and ambulatory monitoring have their place. Ambulatory monitoring provides a profile of blood pressure over a 24-hr period, and shows how the patient responds to the stresses of daily life. Home monitoring provides the most convenient method for assessing changes of blood pressure over time. The two techniques are thus complementary.

REFERENCES

1. Ayman D, Goldshine AD. Blood pressure determinations by patients with essential hypertension: The difference between clinic and home readings before treatment. *Am J Med Sci* 1940;200:465–470.
2. Mancia G, Bertinieri G, Grassi G, Parati G, Pomidossi G, Ferrari A, Gregorini L, Zanchetti A. Effects of blood pressure measurement by the doctor on patient's blood pressure and heart rate. *Lancet* 1983;2:695–697.
3. Mancia G, Parati G, Pomidossi G, Grassi G, Casadei R, Zanchetti A. Alerting reaction and rise in blood pressure during measurement by physician and nurse. *Hypertension* 1987;9:209–215.
4. Pickering TG, James GD, Boddie C, Harshfield GA, Blank S, Laragh JH. How common is white coat hypertension? *JAMA* 1988;259:225–228.
5. Kleinert HD, Harshfield GA, Pickering TG, Devereux RB, Sullivan PA, Marion RM, Mallory WK, Laragh JH. What is the value of home blood pressure measurement in patients with mild hypertension? *Hypertension* 1984;6:574–578.

6. Carey RM, Reid RA, Ayers CR, Lunch SS, McLain WL, Vaughan ED. The Charlottesville blood-pressure survey: value of repeated blood pressure measurements. *JAMA* 1976;236:847–851.
7. Watson RDS, Lamb R, Young MA, Stallard TJ, Davies P, Littler WA. Variation in cuff blood pressure in untreated outpatients with mild hypertension—implications for initiating antihypertensive treatment. *J Hypertens* 1987; 5:207–211.
8. Gordon T, Sorlie P, Kannel WB. Problems in the assessment of blood pressure: the Framingham study. *Int J Epidemiol* 1976;5:327–334.
9. Australian National Blood Pressure Study Management Committee. Untreated mild hypertension. *Lancet* 1982;1:185–191.
10. Medical Research Council Working Party. MRC trial of treatment in mild hypertension: principal results. *Br Med J* 1985;291:97–104.
11. Van Loo JM, Peer PG, Thien TA. Twenty-five minutes between blood pressure readings: the influence on prevalence rates of isolated systolic hypertension. *J Hypertens* 1986;4:631–635.
12. Shimada K, Ogura H, Sadakane N, Kawamoto A, Matsubayashi K, Ozawa T. Within visit blood pressure changes in outpatient clinic. *Hypertension* 1987; 10:465–466.
13. Fagan TC, Conrad KA, Mayshar PV, Mackie MJ, Hagaman RM. Single versus triplicate measurements of blood pressure and heart rate. *Hypertension* 1988;11:282–284.
14. Pickering TG. *Ambulatory monitoring and blood pressure variability*. London: Science Press, 1991.
15. Waeber B, Jacob des Combes B, Porchet M, Biollaz U, Schaller M-D, Brunner HR. Ambulatory blood pressure recording to identify hypertensive patients who truly need therapy. *J Chron Dis* 1984;37:55–57.
16. Corcoran AC, Dustan HP, Page IH. The evaluation of antihypertensive procedures, with particular reference to their effects on blood pressure. *Ann Intern Med* 1955;43:1161–1177.
17. Laughlin KD, Sherrard DH, Fisher L. Comparison of clinic and home blood pressure levels in essential hypertension and variables associated with clinic-home differences. *J Chron Dis* 1979;33:197–206.
18. Badskjaer J, Nielsen PE. Clinical experience using home readings in hypertensive subjects (indirect technique). *Acta Med Scand* 1982;Suppl 670:89–95.
19. Laughlin KD, Fisher L, Sherrard DJ. Blood pressure reductions during self-recording of home blood pressure. *Am Heart J* 1979;98:629–634.
20. Kenny RA, Brennan M, O'Malley K, O'Brien E. Blood pressure measurements in borderline hypertension. *J Hypertens* 1987;5(Suppl 5):S483–S485.
21. James GD, Pickering TG, Yee LS, Harshfield GA, Riva S, Laragh JH. The reproducibility of average ambulatory, home, and clinic pressures. *Hypertension* 1988;11:545–549.
22. Welin L, Svardsudd K, Tibblin G. Home blood pressure measurements—feasibility and results compared to office measurements. *Acta Med Scand* 1982;211:275–279.
23. Beckman M, Panfilov V, Sivertsson R, Sannerstedt R, Anderson O. Blood pressure and heart rate recordings at home and at the clinic. *Acta Med Scand* 1981;210:97–102.
24. Julius S, Ellis CN, Pascual AV, Matice M, Hansson L, Hunyor SN, Sandler

LN. Home blood pressure determination. Value in borderline ("labile") hypertension. *JAMA* 1974;229:663–666.
25. Schneider RH, Egan BM, Johnson EH. Anger and anxiety in borderline hypertension. *Psychosom Med* 1986;48:242–248.
26. Pickering TG, Friedman R. The white coat effect: a neglected role for behavioral factors in hypertension. In: Schneiderman N et al., eds. *Stress, coping, and disease*. Hillsdale, NJ: Erlbaum, 1991.
27. Rostrup M, Kjeldsen SE, Eide I. Awareness of hypertension increases blood pressure and sympathetic responses to cold pressor test. *J Hypertens* 1990; 3:912–917.
28. Engel BT, Baarder KR, Glasgow MS. Behavioral treatment of high blood pressure 1. Analyses of intra- and interdaily variations of blood pressure during a one-month, baseline period. *Psychosom Med* 1981;43:255–270.
29. Pieper C, Schnall PL, Warren K, Pickering TG. Unpublished results.
30. Fagan TC, Konrad KA, Mar JH, Nelson L. Effects of meals on hemodynamics: implications for antihypertensive drug studies. *Clin Pharmacol Ther* 1986;39:255–260.
31. Freestone S, Ramsey LE. Effect of coffee and cigarette smoking on the blood pressure of untreated and diuretic-treated hypertensive patients. *Am J Med* 1982;73:348–353.
32. Gould BA, Dieso HA, Horniung R, Altman DG, Cashman PMM, Raftery EB. Assessment of the accuracy and role of self-recorded blood pressures in the management of hypertension. *Br Med J* 1982;285:1691–1694.
33. Veerman D, Van Montfrans GA, Karemaker J, Wieling W. Inflating one's own cuff does not increase self-recorded blood pressure. *J Hypertens* 1988; 6(Suppl 4):S77–S78.
34. Veerman D, Van Montfrans GA, Wieling W. Effects of cuff inflation on self-recorded blood pressure. *Lancet* 1990;335:451–453.
35. Pickering TG, Cvetkovski B, James GD. An evaluation of electronic recorders for self-monitoring of blood pressure. *J Hypertens* 1986;4(Suppl 5):S328–S330.
36. Leth A, Christau B, Schnohr P, Bruun NE, Muller L. Testing of equipment for home blood pressure reading. *Acta Med Scand* 1982;Suppl 670:85–88.
37. Steiner R, Lüscher T, Boerlin H-J, Siegenthaler W, Vetter W. Clinical evaluation of semiautomatic blood pressure devices for self-recording. *J Hypertens* 1985;3(Suppl 1):23–25.
38. Hunt JC, Frohlich ED, Moser M, Roccella EJ, Keighley EA. Devices used for self-measurement of blood pressure. Revised statement of the National High Blood Pressure Education Program. *Arch Intern Med* 1985;145:2231–2234.
39. O'Brien D, Petrie JC, Littler WA, DeSwiet M. Standards for blood pressure measurement devices. *Br Med J* 1987;294:1245–1246.
40. Shepard DS. Reliability of blood pressure measurements: implications for designing and evaluating programs to control hypertension. *J Chron Dis* 1981; 34:191–209.
41. Editorial. Home blood-pressure recording. *Lancet* 1975;1:259–260.
42. Padfield PL, Lindsay BA, McLaren JA, Pirie A, Rademaker M. Changing relation between home and clinic blood-pressure measurements: do home measurements predict clinic hypertension? *Lancet* 1987;2:322–324.
43. Menard J, Serrurier D, Bautier P, Plouin P-F, Corvol P. Crossover design to

test antihypertensive drugs with self-recorded blood pressure. *Hypertension* 1988;11:153–159.

44. Cottier C, Julius S, Gajendragadlear SV, Schork MA. Usefulness of home BP determination in treating borderline hypertension. *JAMA* 1978;248:535–558.
45. Gould BA, Hornung RS, Kieso H, Cashman PMM, Raftery EB. An evaluation of self-recorded blood pressure during drug trials. *Hypertension* 1986; 8:267–271.
46. Ibrahim MM, Tarazi RC, Dustan HP, Gifford RW. Electrocardiogram in evaluation of resistance to antihypertensive therapy. *Arch Intern Med* 1977; 137:1125–1129.
47. Gordon RD, Pawsey CGK, O'Halloran MW, Abbott ML, Wilson LL, Silverstone H. Use of home-blood-pressure measurement to compare the efficacy of two diuretics. Effects of meclothiazide and furosemide on blood pressure and plasma renin activity and electrolytes. *Med J Aust* 1971;2:565–570.
48. Haynes RB, Sackett DL, Gibson ES, Taylor DW, Hackett BC, Roberts RS, Johnson AL. Improvement of medication compliance in uncontrolled hypertension. *Lancet* 1976;1:1265–1268.
49. Lichtenstein MJ, Sweetnam PM, Elwood PC. Visit frequency for controlled essential hypertension: General practitioner's opinions. *J Fam Pract* 1986; 23:331–336.
50. Parlin DM, Kellett RJ, MacLean DW, et al. The management of hypertension—a study of records in general practice. *J R Coll. Gen Pract* 1979; 29:590–594.
51. Rudneck KV, Sackett DL, Hirst S, Holmas C. Hypertension in a family practice. *Can Med Assoc J* 1977;117:492–497.
52. Perloff D, Gokolow M, Cowan R. The prognostic value of ambulatory blood pressure. *JAMA* 1983;249:2793–2798.
53. Pickering TG, Devereux RB. Ambulatory monitoring of blood pressure as a predictor of cardiovascular risk. *Am Heart J* 1987;114:925–928.
54. Verdecchia P, Bentivoglio M, Provvidenza M, Savino K, Corea L. Reliability of self-recorded arterial pressure in essential hypertension in relation to the stage of the disease. In: Germano G, ed. *Blood pressure recording in the clinical management of hypertension*. Rome: Edizioni L. Pozzi, 1985;40–42.
55. Devereux RB, Pickering TG, Harshfield GA, Kleinert HD, Denby L, Clark L, Pregibon D, Jason M, Kleiner B, Borer JS, Laragh JH. Left ventricular hypertrophy in patients with hypertension. Importance of blood pressure response to regularly recurrent stress. *Circulation* 1983;68:470–476.
56. Pickering TG, Harshfield GA, Kleinert HD, Blank S, Laragh JH. Blood pressure during normal daily activities, sleep, and exercise. *JAMA* 1982;247:992–996.
57. James GD, Cates EM, Pickering TG, Laragh JH. Parity and perceived job stress elevated blood pressure in young normotensive working women. *Am J Hypertens* 1988;1:54A.

Ambulatory Blood Pressure Recording,
edited by H. Brunner and B. Waeber.
Raven Press, Ltd., New York © 1992.

7

Efficacy Assessment of Antihypertensive Therapy

*Bernard Waeber, †Eoin O'Brien, *Edoardo Camenzind, †John Cox, *Jürg Nussberger, and *Hans R. Brunner

**Division of Hypertension, University Hospital, Lausanne, Switzerland, and †Blood Pressure Unit, Beaumont Hospital, Dublin, Ireland*

Accurate blood pressure measurement is crucial for evaluation of antihypertensive therapy. At first glance, this does not seem to be a difficult task. There are, however, several sources of error that may hamper the precise assessment of the blood pressure lowering effect of drugs (35,53). In everyday practice, blood pressure is determined traditionally by the noninvasive auscultatory method based on the principle of arterial occlusion using a forearm cuff. Blood pressure readings obtained by this approach are not always reliable because of potentially important technical inconstancies and observer bias. Another problem is linked with the fact that blood pressure varies spontaneously throughout the day. Moreover, conventionally measured office blood pressures are often only a poor reflection of blood pressure outside of the medical environment.

It is now possible to monitor blood pressure over prolonged periods outside the physician's office either intra-arterially or noninvasively using portable devices (28). It appears relevant, therefore, to review the advantages and the inconveniences of this new way of investigating the efficacy of antihypertensive treatment. This chapter focuses on the experience accumulated over the past few years with the monitoring of ambulatory blood pressure in clinical trials. The usefulness of self-recorded blood pressures as an alternative mode of assessing blood pressure responses in drug studies will also be discussed.

CHARACTERIZATION OF ANTIHYPERTENSIVE THERAPY

The benefits and inconveniences of the various methods of measuring blood pressure are summarized in Table 1.

Casual Office Blood Pressures

The method routinely used to assess the efficacy of antihypertensive drugs has practically not changed over the years. Basically, the blood pressure of a hypertensive patient is evaluated sporadically by a physician using a mercury sphygmomanometer. There are undoubtedly good reasons to do so. The technique of blood pressure measurement is very simple and is therefore well suited to the long-term follow-up of hypertensive patients. Moreover, almost everything known about the beneficial effects of pharmacological blood pressure reduction on the risk of major cardiovascular complications is derived from office blood pressure readings.

It should be stressed, however, that casual blood pressures determined by physicians are not always accurate. Office blood pressure measurements are subject to potentially large observer variations (3). Regular training of physicians involved in the care of hypertensive patients improves the observer performance. The need for training sessions is unfortunately not often perceived by the physi-

TABLE 1. *Benefits and inconveniences of the various methods of measuring blood pressure*

	Casual office or clinic BP	Invasive ambulatory BP	Noninvasive ambulatory BP	Home self-recorded BP
Accuracy	+	+ + +	+ +	+
Reproducibility	+	+ +	+ +	+
"White-coat" effect	+ +	−	−	−
Observer bias	+ +	−	−	+ +
Potential side effects	−	+	−	−
Correlation with cardiovascular risk	+	+ + +	+ + +	+ +
Cost	+	+ + +	+ +	−

cians. To avoid inaccurate blood pressure measurements, several conditions are required as proposed by the World Health Organization and the International Society of Hypertension (34,56). For instance, one has to recall that instruments used to measure blood pressure have to be calibrated regularly, a precaution that is taken only seldom by practitioners. Another problem is the widespread habit of physicians to approximate blood pressure readings by choosing preferentially as last digit either 0 or 5. This is illustrated by the findings of a recent controlled trial conducted in general practice in which more than 90% of blood pressure readings were expressed by 0 or 5 (47). The use of automatic machines to measure blood pressure is expected to reduce observer bias. Of course, this is assuming that the device has been validated satisfactorily and is operated properly. An alternative approach to measure blood pressure in clinical trials is the use of the random-zero sphygmomanometer (38). This device has the advantage over the standard mercury sphygmomanometer of leaving the observer blind to the actual blood pressure level until it has been recorded. On the other hand, it has the shortcoming of giving systematically lower readings than the standard mercury sphygmomanometer.

Of these factors, the one most likely to influence the levels of office blood pressure is the doctor-patient relationship. The presence of a physician may lead to transient, potentially large blood pressure increases of a basically unpredictable magnitude (14,21, 29,41). It is still not clear why the pressor effect of the physician is more pronounced in some individuals than in others. What is sure is that this phenomenon also exists, albeit to a lesser degree, when blood pressure is measured by a nurse. The alerting response provoked by the presence of a physician tends to decrease with time, making it mandatory to have repeated blood pressure measurements before making a therapeutic decision (37,51). Up to six visits may be needed for full evaluation of office blood pressure. However, the magnitude of the rise in blood pressure occurring in the physician's office usually does not disappear entirely during long-term follow-up.

Another aspect to be considered is the time of the day at which office blood pressure readings are obtained. Physiologically, blood pressure reaches its highest level at midmorning, to fall thereafter throughout the day to its nadir in sleep with a rise again before waking (27). This circadian pattern of blood pressure variation should ideally be taken into account when ascertaining at the physician's office the blood pressure lowering effect of drugs. In addition, the levels of blood pressure measured at different moments of the day might depend more or less on the time of drug administration. This is a serious drawback to the use of office blood pressure measurements for assessment of the efficacy of antihypertensive therapy. It is generally not feasible to plan a series of visits on the same day in order to establish a blood pressure profile.

Home Blood Pressure Measurements

Complementary information on blood pressure levels prevailing outside the physician's office can be obtained by asking the patients or their relatives to measure blood pressure at home. The technique can be learned accurately by most people (24). One of the common objections to self-measurement of blood pressure is that patients might be made anxious by knowledge of their own blood pressure. This, however, does not seem to represent a true problem. Blood pressure determined at home tends indeed to decrease while patients become habituated to the conditions of measurement (25).

Self-measured blood pressures seem to be more representative of cardiovascular risk than office blood pressure (see chapter by Pickering). The equipment is often more or less automated, but there are many self-inflatable devices available. Why then not extend the application of this technique to every patient? The major concerns regard the accuracy and the potential misuse of the instruments, mainly because of a lack of adequate instruction. Improper calibration of the devices may also represent a problem (35,36). In this respect the accuracy of home sphygmomanometers has been evaluated in a population survey. The results demonstrated that 64% of the blood pressure measuring machines were accurate within ± 2 mmHg, and an additional 26% within ± 3 to 6 mmHg (20). Also to be taken into consideration is the fact that many patients are reluctant to measure their blood pressure at home. Finally, not all doctors accept the value of home blood pressure measurements.

Continuous Monitoring of Intra-Arterial Pressure

If the intra-arterial technique of ambulatory measurement still represents the gold standard, it has nevertheless the disadvantage of being invasive, and consequently it is not suitable for routine assessment of blood pressure in clinical trials (Table 1). However, much knowledge can be gained by monitoring blood pressure invasively. For instance, this mode of blood pressure measurement is particularly valid to study the impact of antihypertensive drugs on "beat-to-beat" blood pressure and heart rate variability (27,28). This is also true for the precise evaluation of blood pressure during sleep and strenuous physical exercise (16).

Noninvasive Ambulatory Blood Pressure Monitoring

Ambulatory blood pressure profiles can now be recorded noninvasively by a number of compact, portable devices (36,48,55). These blood pressure measuring apparatuses are either semiautomatic, requiring the participation of the patients, or fully automatic, with the cuff being inflated at preset intervals. The use of recorders that have to be activated by the patients is limited to the daytime period, whereas automated machines allow whole-day blood pressure monitoring. The recording of ambulatory blood pressure using such equipment is very appealing, particularly for the evaluation of the effectiveness of antihypertensive therapy when it is possible to perform repeat recordings in the same patient. The modern devices provide accurate blood pressure readings. The ambulatory blood pressure levels appear to be meaningful since they tend to correlate better with the risk of developing a cardiovascular complication than office blood pressures (see Perloff and Sokolow). However, the lack of well-established criteria of normalcy for ambulatory blood pressure remains a problem. Another disadvantage is the high cost of the blood pressure monitoring systems.

COMPARISON BETWEEN OFFICE, HOME, AND AMBULATORY BLOOD PRESSURE RECORDINGS

The three methods of measuring blood pressure have been compared in the same patients in several studies (13, 22–24,30). Ambulatory recorded pressures are on the average consistently lower than readings taken by a doctor. Home blood pressures are usually somewhere in between, closer to blood pressure levels obtained by ambulatory monitoring than to office blood pressures.

The validity of one mode of blood pressure determination in characterizing the effectiveness of antihypertensive therapy depends greatly on the reproducibility of the measurements. One might expect blood pressure levels recorded under variable circumstances to be less reproducible than office and home blood pressures, the two latter being collected in relatively standardized settings. In fact, the average of daytime recorded pressures is well reproducible over periods of several months, both in normotensive subjects and hypertensive patients (21,22,52). In one study, the reproducibility of ambulatory blood pressure recordings appeared to be better than that of office measurements and similar to that of home readings (22). Figure 1 illustrates the results of a study aimed at comparing the efficacy of two drug regimens (42). The magnitude of the blood pressure response to both treatments was found to correlate better over a period of a few weeks when calculated from ambulatory rather than office readings. Most probably this phenomenon is due to the large number of measurements obtained during an ambulatory recording. The mean of all readings is less sensitive to extreme blood pressure fluctuations.

UNPREDICTABILITY OF HOME READINGS AND AMBULATORY BLOOD PRESSURE RECORDINGS

As already stated, a factor complicating therapeutic decision-making in the individual subject is the difference between office blood pressures and those determined at home or recorded away from the doctor during usual daytime activities.

As shown in Table 2, the difference between home and office

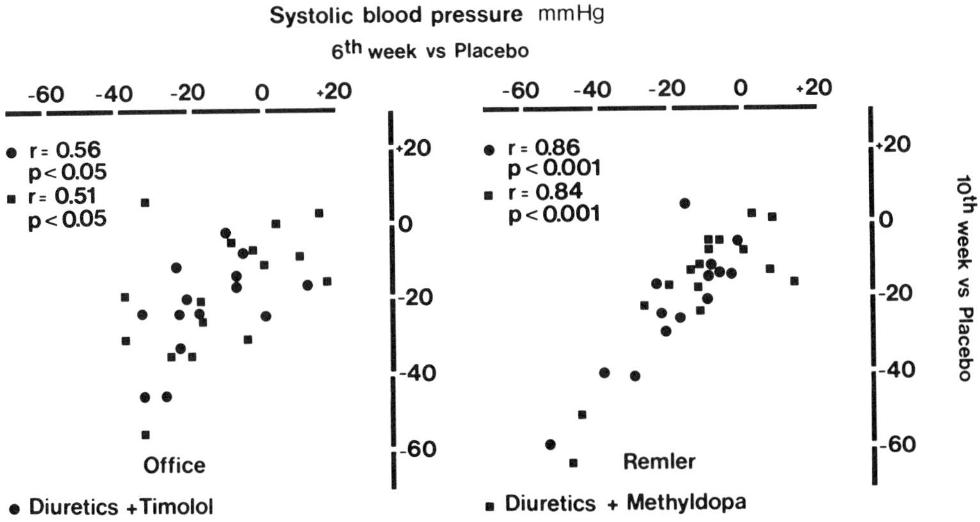

FIG. 1. Relationship between the magnitude of the systolic blood pressure responses to a 6-week treatment (diuretics combined with timolol or methyldopa) assessed either conventionally by a doctor at his office or using an ambulatory blood pressure recorder. (From ref. 42, with permission.)

pressures or ambulatory recorded pressures is so wide that at a given point it becomes impossible to derive with some confidence one type of pressure from the other (23). This is also true for the difference between home pressures and ambulatory pressures recorded intra-arterially. Here again, the agreement between the two sets of blood pressure levels is too weak to allow any predictions in the individual patient (18).

The same kind of observation has been made comparing office with ambulatory pressures recorded with a portable device. For instance, ambulatory systolic and diastolic pressures were found lower than corresponding office pressures by approximately 10 mmHg in unselected, untreated subjects (21). However, it was not possible in any given subject to predict the level of ambulatory pressure from blood pressure readings taken by a physician. In some subjects, differences of over 30 mmHg were observed between the two kinds of pressures. Alternatively, ambulatory recorded blood pressures were higher than office pressures in approximately 10% of the subjects.

TABLE 2. *Casual office, home, and ambulatory recorded blood pressures (mmHg) measured on three occasions at 2-week intervals in patients with borderline hypertension (n = 19)*

	Office		Home		Ambulatory	
Controls	SBP	DBP	SBP	DBP	SBP	DBP
1	159 ± 13	99 ± 9	148 ± 13	94 ± 12	139 ± 15	88 ± 10
2	156 ± 10	97 ± 10	148 ± 13	94 ± 13	142 ± 14	92 ± 9
3	153 ± 15	97 ± 14	144 ± 15	94 ± 13	136 ± 16	90 ± 9
	NS	NS	NS	NS	NS	NS

SBP, systolic blood pressure; DBP, diastolic blood pressure; NS, no significant difference between recording intervals for each technique; results are given as means ± SD.

Major differences between ambulatory recorded and office blood pressures were also noticed in hypertensive patients, whether treated or not (41,48). An example is given in Fig. 2. Seventeen patients with uncomplicated essential hypertension were given either the beta-blocker betaxolol or the calcium antagonist verapamil for two consecutive 6-week periods. The sequence of treatment phases was randomly allocated and a 2-week washout period preceded each treatment. Blood pressures measured by a physician are plotted against the difference between office blood pressure readings and the corresponding mean ambulatory recorded pressures. Office pressures were markedly higher than recorded pressures in most patients, and differences exceeding 20 mmHg systolic and 10 mmHg diastolic were common. This was the case at the time the patients were untreated as well as at the end of each treatment phase. Notwithstanding, some patients exhibited a lower blood pressure in the physician's presence than during customary daily activity. Once again, the most striking finding was the impossibility of predicting the magnitude of the difference between office and

FIG. 2. Comparison between office blood pressure and the difference between office blood pressure (BP) readings and the corresponding mean of daytime ambulatory recorded pressures. Both office and recorded pressures were determined at the end of a 4-week washout and after completion of a 4-week treatment with betaxolol and verapamil. The *upper* and *lower panels* correspond to systolic and diastolic pressures, respectively. (From ref. 48.)

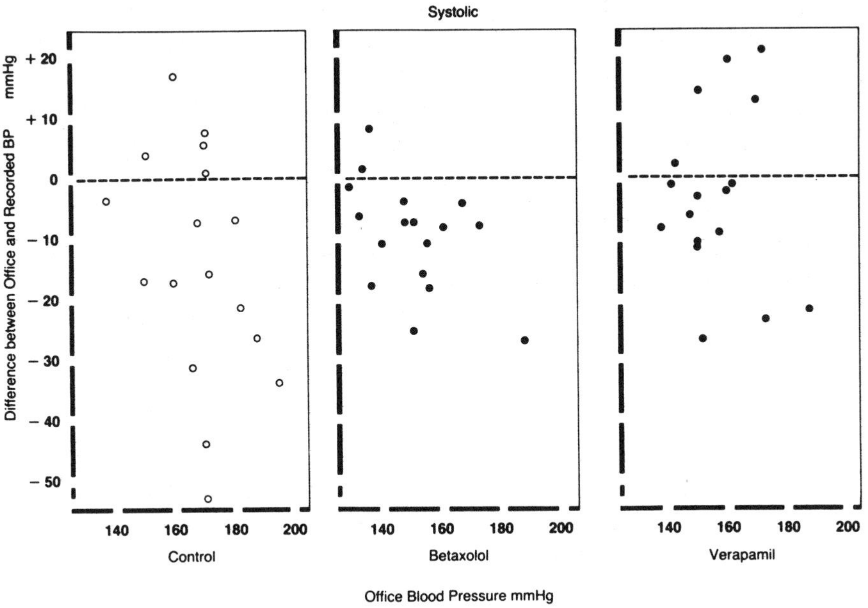
Systolic
Difference between Office and Recorded BP mmHg
+ 20
+ 10
0
– 10
– 20
– 30
– 40
– 50
140 160 180 200
Control
140 160 180 200
Betaxolol
140 160 180 200
Verapamil
Office Blood Pressure mmHg

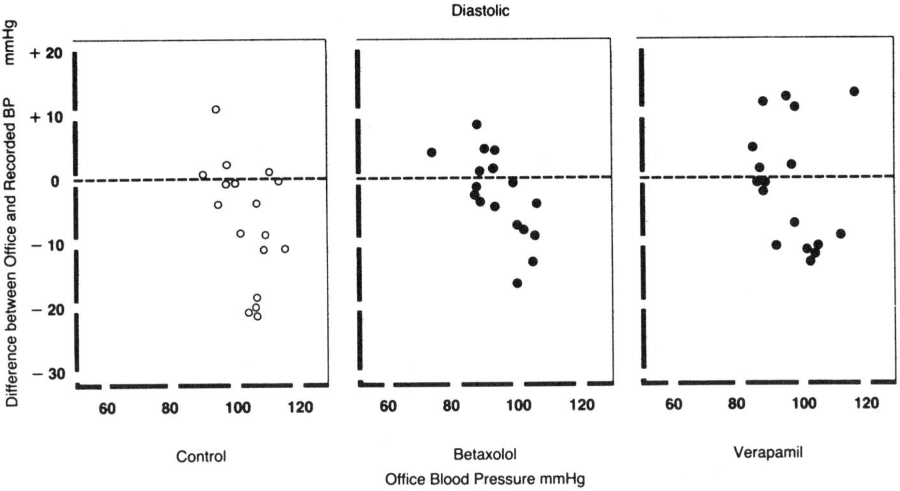
Diastolic
Difference between Office and Recorded BP mmHg
+ 20
+ 10
0
– 10
– 20
– 30
60 80 100 120
Control
60 80 100 120
Betaxolol
60 80 100 120
Verapamil
Office Blood Pressure mmHg

ambulatory recorded blood pressures based on the physician's blood pressure measurement. This observation is in agreement with the experience of other investigators who have used the intra-arterial route to monitor ambulatory blood pressure (14,18,29). The average pressor response to the physician tends to remain on the same order of magnitude when assessed over a few months in a sample of an unselected population (21). However, the reproducibility of individual responses seems too poor in hypertensives to permit accurate prediction in a given patient (11). Clinically relevant is the fact that the blood pressure rise occurring when encountering a physician seems to be unaffected by antihypertensive therapies with different mechanisms of action (11,48).

HOME AND AMBULATORY RECORDED BLOOD PRESSURES AS A MEANS OF AVOIDING OVERTREATMENT OF HYPERTENSIVE PATIENTS

Therapeutic decisions are most difficult in the hypertensive patient free of target organ damage and exhibiting only modestly elevated blood pressures. In such a patient, the factor determining ordinarily the need for treatment is usually the level of office blood pressure per se. It is therefore mandatory not to initiate treatment until blood pressure elevation has been confirmed on a number of visits (51). Asking the patient to measure his or her blood pressure at home may help to recognize those patients whose blood pressure is only elevated at the physician's office (36). For the same purpose, increasing use is being made of ambulatory blood pressure monitoring (36).

Assessment of blood pressure away from the clinical setting seems particularly justified in patients with borderline hypertension. Table 2 shows as an example the values of blood pressures measured in such patients by three different methods on three occasions at 2-week intervals (23). Conventional blood pressure readings obtained by a physician gave levels that were higher than ambulatory measurements, with self-recorded measurements falling between the two. Looking at the average and the standard deviation of daytime ambulatory recorded blood pressures, it is apparent that a number of patients had systolic and diastolic levels well below 140 and 90 mmHg, respectively, during the monitoring periods. This is in close agreement with previous observations made using continuous recording of direct arterial pressure in unrestricted patients (14).

This raises the problem of how to manage untreated patients who are hypertensive according to office blood pressures but who have normal blood pressures from the morning to the evening when pursuing their everyday activities. In other words, whereas antihypertensive drugs may lower the office pressure, it does not necessarily follow that they will reduce blood pressures prevailing outside the physician's office. This question has been addressed in the analysis of a recent trial aimed at comparing the blood pressure lowering effect of two antihypertensive drugs in untreated patients with essential hypertension (50). Figure 3 depicts the results observed with betaxolol. After 4 weeks of treatment, this agent did not reduce ambulatory blood pressure consistently in patients who had already low ambulatory blood pressures at the beginning of the study. The same observations were made with verapamil (not shown). Thus,

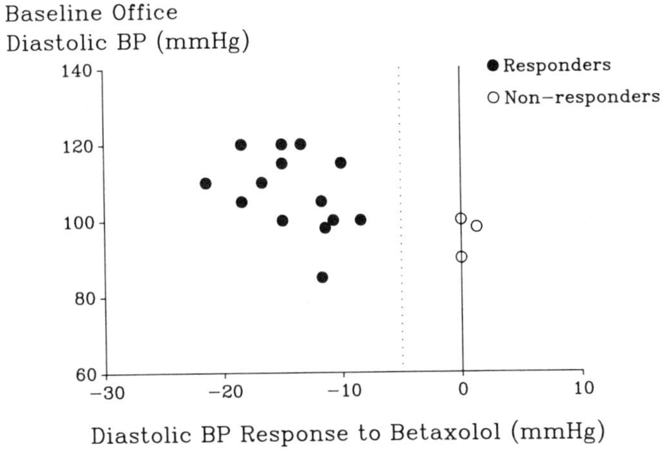

FIG. 3. Relationship between the changes in diastolic blood pressure induced by betaxolol and the pretreatment blood pressure levels. Patients were considered responders when the magnitude of the drug-induced blood pressure fall was larger than 5 mmHg.

diagnosis of hypertension based solely on office blood pressure values may lead to overdiagnosis of hypertension and overtreatment of a nonnegligible fraction of the population.

Home and ambulatory blood pressure monitoring can also be recommended in the evaluation of patients with treatment-resistant hypertension (26,32,39). In 38 chronically treated hypertensive patients who continued to exhibit abnormally high office blood pressures, ambulatory recorded blood pressures were, on the average, lower by almost 30 mmHg for systolic and 15 mmHg for diastolic than corresponding blood pressures determined in the doctor's office (41). In most patients, ambulatory blood pressures could not be predicted from office blood pressure readings.

That one should take into account blood pressure measured outside the physician's office when trying to decide on a therapeutic strategy is also suggested by the experience obtained in elderly hypertensive patients who underwent ambulatory blood pressure monitoring because of persistent, abnormally high casual blood pressure levels (office blood pressure ≥160 mmHg for systolic and/or ≥95 mmHg for diastolic) (45). Several interesting features emerged from the retrospective analysis of the therapeutic decisions that had been based on the results of the ambulatory blood pressure profiles. First, patients who were considered to have normal ambulatory pressures (<160/90 mmHg) tended to have decreasing office blood pressures during the 4- to 8-month follow-up. The blood pressure reduction occurred even though previously untreated patients remained without antihypertensive treatment and previously treated patients were maintained on an unchanged regimen (Fig. 4, upper panel). The most likely explanations for this finding are a progressive familiarization of the patient with his doctor and regression to the mean. Nevertheless, even in these patients, office blood pressures remained higher than ambulatory recorded blood pressures throughout the observation period. In sharp contrast, those patients who were still hypertensive during their usual daily activities exhibited ambulatory blood pressure levels that were barely lower than office blood pressures (Fig. 4, lower panel). In these patients, starting or modifying antihypertensive treatment markedly decreased office blood pressures. In fact, the degree of blood pressure control obtained at

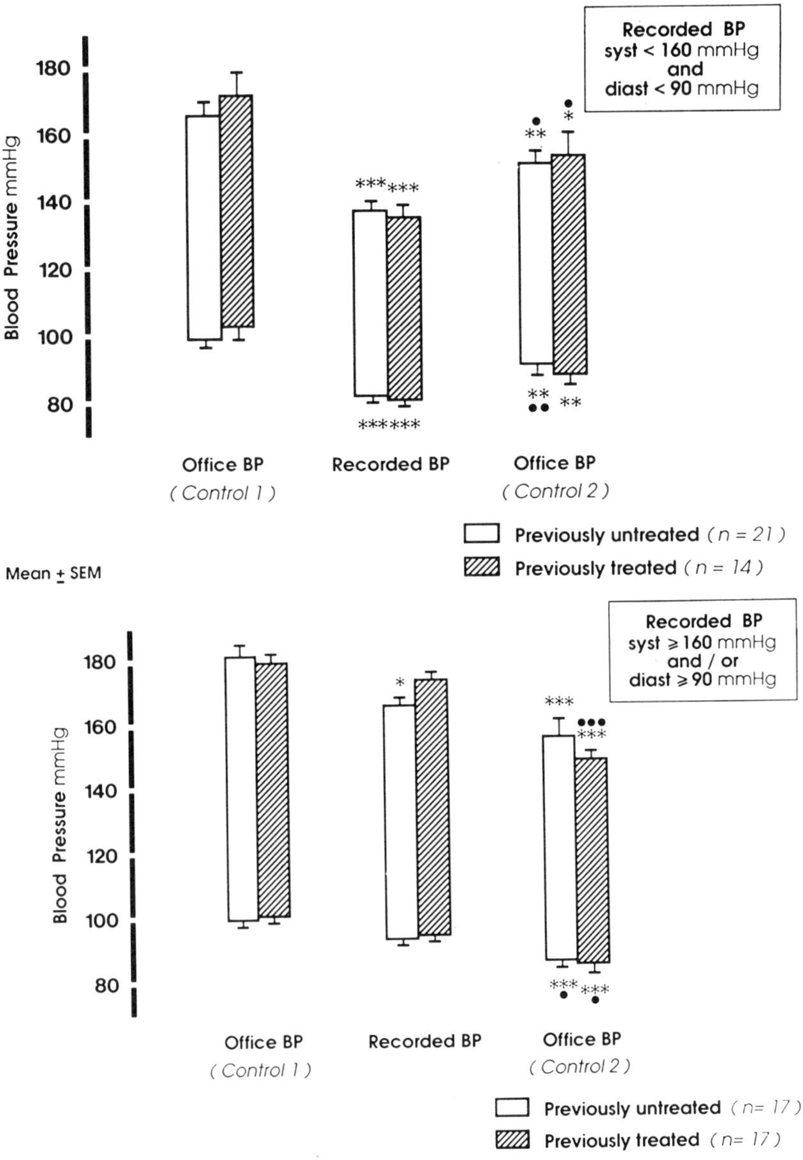

FIG. 4. Blood pressure (BP) levels (mean ± SEM) measured by a doctor in his office at a 4- to 8-month interval in elderly hypertensive patients with either normal (*upper panel*) or abnormally high blood pressure (*lower panel*) during ambulatory blood pressure monitoring. **p*<.05, ***p*<.05, ****p*<.001 vs Control *1; *p*<.05, ***p*<.01, ****p*<.001, vs recorded blood pressure.

the physician's office at the end of the follow-up was very similar in those patients who at the outset had high pressures and in those with normal ambulatory pressures.

The most striking results came from a prospective study in which ambulatory blood pressure was monitored in 34 hypertensive patients with an office diastolic pressure of 95 mmHg or more despite antihypertensive therapy (49). Treatment was adjusted in these patients with the aim of reducing office diastolic pressure to 90 mmHg or less within 3 months. Ambulatory blood pressures were monitored at the beginning and the end of the study, but the results of these recordings were not made available to the physicians until completion of the trial. At the outset of the study, recorded ambulatory diastolic pressure was 90 mmHg or less in half the patients (Group A) and above 90 mmHg in the other half (Group B). The office and ambulatory diastolic blood pressures of these two groups of patients were depicted in Fig. 5 (upper panel for Group A and lower panel for Group B). Systolic pressures followed the same pattern as diastolic blood pressures in both groups (not shown). Differences in baseline office blood pressures between the two groups were small and only the diastolic but not the systolic pressure was significantly higher in Group B. On the last assessment at the physician's office, there was no significant difference in diastolic pressures between the two groups. During the final ambulatory blood pressure recording, however, diastolic pressures were still significantly lower in Group A than in Group B. The target office diastolic pressure of 90 mmHg or less was achieved in 11 patients of Group A and 7 of Group B. In Group A patients, the change in antihypertensive therapy significantly reduced office blood pressure. No significant modification of ambulatory blood pressure was seen at the same time. In Group B patients, diastolic pressure fell significantly during the trial, not only when measured by the physician, but also when recorded in the ambulatory patient. From these data, one can draw the conclusion that intensifying the therapy of hypertensive patients who have a normal ambulatory blood pressure may result in overtreatment without real gain in blood pressure control.

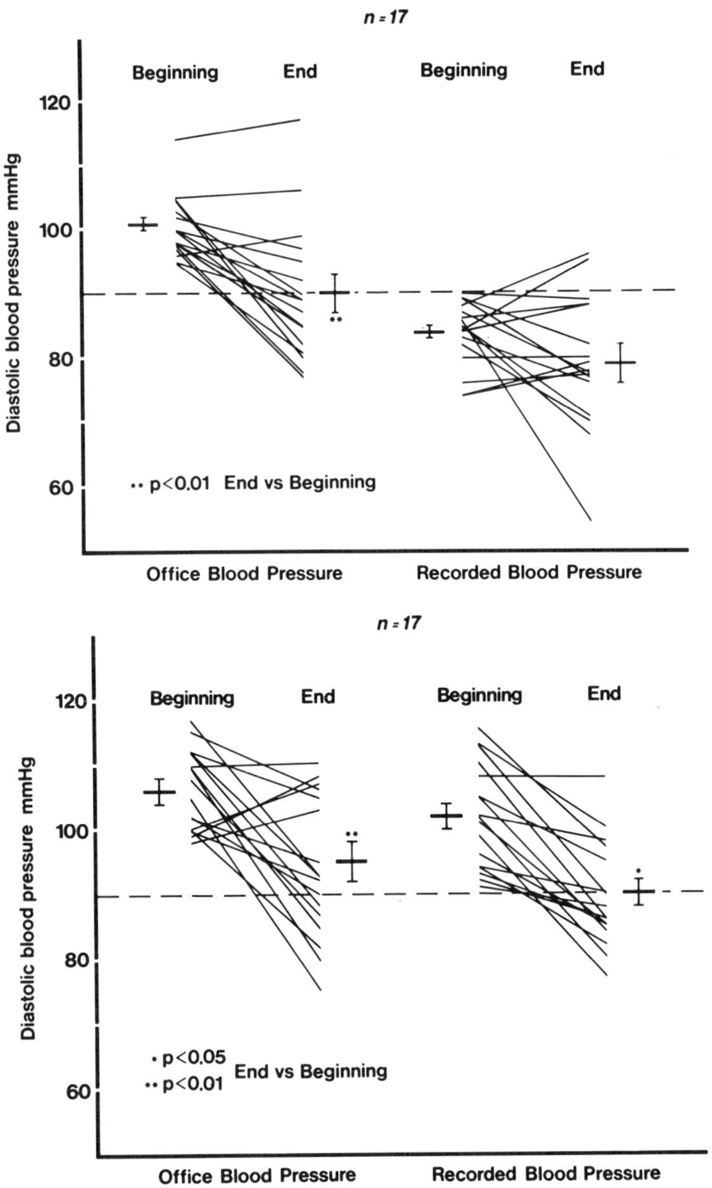

FIG. 5. Office and abmulatory diastolic blood pressures at the beginning and the end of the study in patients with a diastolic pressure ≤ 90 mmHg (Group A, *upper panel*) or > 90 mmHg (Group B, *lower panel*) during initial ambulatory blood pressure monitoring. Means ± SEM **p*<.05, ***p*<.01, end vs beginning.

ASSESSMENT OF BLOOD PRESSURE IN THERAPEUTIC TRIALS

Utility of Blood Pressure Readings Obtained by Self-Determination

There are only scanty reports on the use of self-recorded blood pressures during drug trials (15,17,23,31,33). In one study aimed at comparing the efficacy of the alpha-blocking agent prazosin and the calcium antagonist verapamil, the reductions in blood pressure produced by the antihypertensive treatment were of similar magnitude when assessed intra-arterially (23/19 ± 12/10 mmHg, mean ± SD) and noninvasively at home (24/16 ± 18/7 mmHg) (17). However, intraindividual blood pressure changes obtained with the two techniques showed poor agreement. Home blood pressure monitoring was therefore considered suitable for estimating the blood pressure lowering effect of a drug in a group of patients, but not for characterizing the blood pressure response in a given subject.

Other investigators have performed a within-patient trial with the goal of measuring blood pressure both at the clinic and at home (33). The test agents consisted of the beta-blocking agent oxprenolol and a combination of diuretics (chlorthalidone and triamterene). In comparison with placebo, the diuretics lowered blood pressure by 14/3 ± 11/9 mmHg (mean ± SD) at the clinic and by 9/5 ± 11/7 mmHg at home. The corresponding values for the beta-blocker were 14/8 ± 14/7 and 5/3 ± 12/9 mmHg. The fact that oxprenolol seemed more effective at the clinic than at home was attributed to a possible blunting effect of the beta-blocker on the arousal response that occurs during blood pressure measurement by a doctor. A major effort was made in this study to get an extensive statistical analysis. There was less dispersion of the data when using home than clinic blood pressure measurements, indicating that the statistical power of a trial can be improved by asking patients to monitor their blood pressure at home.

Another important aspect to be pointed out is the impact of blood pressure self-measurement on patient adherence to treatment (10). Blood pressure recording at home during drug trials may indeed increase compliance with antihypertensive therapy.

Value of Ambulatory Blood Pressure Monitoring

Placebo Effect

An important issue in drug trials is the placebo effect on blood pressure. Though not confirmed in every study, the evidence overwhelmingly suggests that administration of a placebo significantly reduces office blood pressure. It is therefore widely accepted that a trial planned to evaluate precisely the antihypertensive efficacy of an active compound should include a placebo phase. It now appears that the administration of a placebo only lowers the blood pressure readings taken by a physician, and not ambulatory blood pressures monitored intra-arterially (19). More recent observations based on noninvasive intermittent ambulatory blood pressure recordings support this view (1,8,9,40,54). An example is given in Table 3. In this study, a significant blood pressure reduction was noticed only at the physician's office during a 4-week placebo period (9). Thus, assessment of antihypertensive efficacy of drugs by utilizing ambulatory blood pressure monitors might render the use of placebo in therapeutic trials unnecessary. Of course, placebo-controlled trials remain of critical importance for the evaluation of the real incidence of adverse effects.

TABLE 3. *Blood pressure before and after placebo (means ± SEM) in 46 hypertensive patients*

	Baseline	Placebo
Systolic (mmHg)		
Clinic	174.6 ± 8.1	161.8 ± 7.6[a]
Ambulatory	158.3 ± 6.8	154.6 ± 7.1
Diastolic (mmHg)		
Clinic	109.8 ± 3.9	104.2 ± 4.1[a]
Ambulatory	103.0 ± 3.6	101.8 ± 4.1

[a] $p<.001$ as compared with baseline.

Statistical Power

In most therapeutic trials, patients are seen sporadically at the physician's office, and only a very few blood pressure readings are available for analysis. Ambulatory blood pressure monitoring is clearly advantageous in that it provides a substantial number of blood pressure values that can be averaged (4,5). This means that the influence of within-subject blood pressure variability is attenuated, thus improving the statistical power. This theoretical consideration is supported by a number of studies. The superiority of multiple readings in estimating the blood pressure lowering effect of drugs is well illustrated by the fact that conventional clinic measurements may fail to detect a significant blood pressure effect, whereas clear-cut blood pressure reductions can be demonstrated by ambulatory recordings. Such a phenomenon is already apparent in trials comprising small numbers of patients. For instance, the administration of a clonidine transdermal therapeutic system to severely hypertensive patients produced a negligible fall in office diastolic blood pressure of 6 mmHg, whereas the ambulatory blood pressure monitoring revealed a highly significant decrease of 21 mmHg (43). Major discrepancies between blood pressure responses assessed in the clinic and corresponding ambulatory recorded blood pressure changes have also been demonstrated in controlled trials. In a comparison of the antihypertensive efficacy of timolol with that of methyldopa in 30 hypertensive patients, office blood pressure readings suggested no difference between the two compounds, whereas ambulatory blood pressure recordings indicated that timolol was significantly more effective in lowering diastolic pressure (42). Also, the alpha-blocking agent trimazosin was found to be equally effective in 22 hypertensive patients as the beta-blocker propranolol when the analysis was based on clinic blood pressure readings (8). However, ambulatory recorded pressures showed that propranolol provided much better results than trimazosin. Interestingly, there also are circumstances in which significant reductions in clinic blood pressure cannot be confirmed by ambulatory blood pressure monitoring (12, 42,49). It may even happen that the clinic blood pressure reduction coincides only with a brief period of blood pressure reduction in the whole ambulatory blood pressure profile (6).

Individualization of Antihypertensive Therapy

The precision gained by ambulatory blood pressure monitoring gives more weight to the observations made in the individual subject. This is very important since drugs acting by different mechanisms may be more or less effective in a given patient. This hypothesis was tested for instance by comparing the antihypertensive effect of a calcium antagonist with that of an angiotensin converting enzyme (ACE) inhibitor (2). Patients with essential hypertension were treated in a randomized crossover trial for two consecutive 6-week periods with either diltiazem or enalapril. The two drugs were equipotent in lowering blood pressure. There was no evidence (Fig. 6) that a good response to one drug excluded a similarly good response to the other. Of note is the fact that each point illustrated in the figure represents the average of 24 blood pressures recorded during the daytime, which strongly strengthens the validity of the observation.

ANALYSIS OF NONINVASIVE AMBULATORY BLOOD PRESSURE RECORDINGS

A common way of presenting the blood pressure recordings is to average all readings (52,53,55). This approach is meaningful only if awake and sleep blood pressures are assessed separately. It is recommended to measure blood pressure at 15- to 30-min intervals during the daytime (46). The average of blood pressures recorded intermittently in such conditions is indeed known to reflect the mean of all beat-to-beat intra-arterial pressures that could be determined continuously during the whole monitoring interval (7). To minimize the influence of artifacts or extreme sample points, nonparametric analysis may be used. For instance, the arithmetical mean can be replaced by the median and the standard deviations by the interquartile ranges.

In addition to the calculation of awake and sleep blood pressures, what is happening in shorter periods within the overall 24-hr profile, for example, in the preawakening period, may be of great interest. However, the reduction of the number of measurements automatically leads to a loss in the statistical power. For instance, it may become really difficult to detect any significant difference when hourly blood pressure changes are considered.

The examination of the 24-hr blood pressure profile also provides

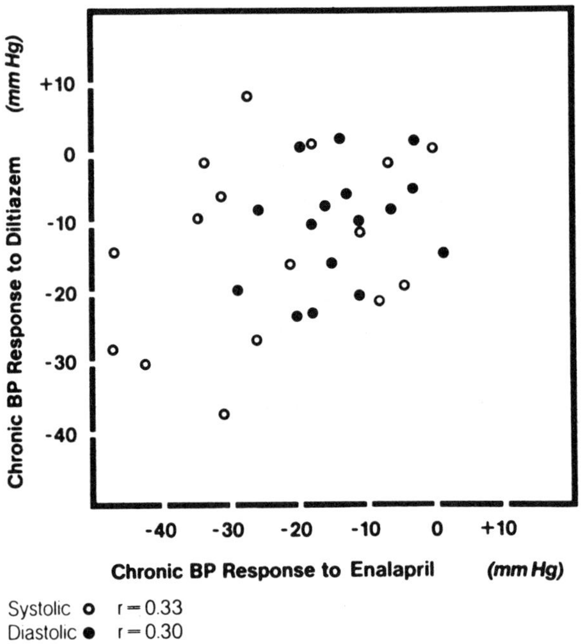

FIG. 6. Relationship between blood pressure responses to 6-week treatments with diltiazem and enalapril. The drugs were administered to 16 patients in a random order according to a crossover design. (From ref. 2.)

the pattern of an antihypertensive effect over the dosing interval. Ambulatory blood pressure recordings are expected to be particularly valuable for the study of the trough and peak periods of efficacy of antihypertensive drugs, permitting assessment of duration of action.

Finally, different mathematical methods have been proposed for the statistical analysis of circadian blood pressure recordings (Cosinor analysis for instance). The practical usefulness of these sophisticated tools of analysis still remains under investigation (44).

CONCLUSIONS

Blood pressures taken by a physician often do not permit estimation of the level of blood pressure prevailing while the patient remains in his usual environment. In the individual patient, the magnitude of the blood pressure changes elicited by the presence of a doctor cannot be predicted. Recording self-measured or ambulatory blood pressure is therefore very attractive for determining the need for antihypertensive therapy in a given patient as well as the quality of blood pressure control achieved by the treatment. Assessment of ambulatory blood pressure in drug trials makes it possible to minimize the number of patients used and may render the planning of a placebo phase unnecessary. Careful analysis of ambulatory blood pressure profiles can also help to define the time course of the blood pressure lowering effect of antihypertensive agents.

ACKNOWLEDGMENTS

This work was supported by grants from the Swiss National Science Foundation and the Cardiovascular Research Foundation.

REFERENCES

1. Berglund G, De Faire U, Castenfors J, Andersson G, Hartford M, Liedholm H, Ljungman S, Thulin T, Wikstrand J. Monitoring 24-hour blood pressure in a drug trial. Evaluation of a non-invasive device. *Hypertension* 1985;7:688–694.
2. Bidiville J, Nussberger J, Waeber G, Porchet M, Waeber B, Brunner HR. Individual responses to converting enzyme inhibitors and calcium antagonists. *Hypertension* 1988;11:166–173.
3. Bruce NG, Shaper AG, Walker M, Wannamethee G. Observer bias in blood pressure studies. *J Hypertens* 1988;6:375–380.
4. Coats AJS, Conway J, Somers VK, Isea JE, Sleight P. Ambulatory pressure monitoring in the assessment of antihypertensive therapy. *Cardiovasc Drug Ther* 1989;3:303-311.
5. Conway J, Johnston J, Coats A, Somers V, Sleight P. The use of ambulatory blood pressure monitoring to improve the accuracy and reduce the numbers of subjects in clinical trials of antihypertensive agents. *J Hypertens* 1988;6:111–116.
6. Cox JP, O'Boyle CA, Mee F, Kelly J, Atkins N, Coakley D, O'Brien E, O'Malley K. The antihypertensive efficacy of verapamil in the elderly evaluated by ambulatory blood pressure. *J Hum Hypertens* 1988;2:41–47.
7. Di Rienzo M, Grassi G, Pedotti A, Mancia G. Continuous versus intermittent blood pressure measurements in estimating 24 hour average blood pressure. *Hypertension* 1983;5:264–269.
8. Drayer JIM, Weber MA, De Young JL, Brewer DD. Long-term blood pressure monitoring in the evaluation of antihypertensive therapy. *Arch Intern Med* 1983;143:898–901.

9. Dupont AG, Van der Niepen P, Six O. Placebo does not lower ambulatory blood pressure. *Br J Clin Pharmacol* 1987;24:106–109.
10. Edmonds D, Foerster E, Groth H, Greminger P, Siegenthaler W, Vetter W. Does self-measurement of blood pressure improve patient compliance in hypertension? *J Hypertens* 1985;3(Suppl 1):31–34.
11. Elijovich F, Laffer CL. Magnitude, reproducibility, and components of the pressor response to the clinic. *Hypertension* 1990;15(suppl 1):161–165.
12. Enström I, Thulen T, Lindholm L. A plea for more comprehensive blood pressure measurements when evaluating drug treatment of hypertension. *J Hypertens* 1988;6:959–964.
13. Flapan AD, Stewart SE, McDougal F, Padfield PL. Is self home monitoring of blood pressure as good as 24-hour ambulatory monitoring? *J Hypertens* 1987; 5(suppl 5):491–493.
14. Floras JS, Jones JV, Hassan MO, Osikowska B, Sever PS, Sleight P. Cuff and ambulatory pressure in subjects with essential hypertension. *Lancet* 1981; 2:107–109.
15. Gordon RD, Pawsey CGK, O'Halloran MW, Abbott ML, Wilson LL, Silverstone H. Use of home-blood pressure measurement to compare the efficacy of two diuretics. Effects of methyclothiazide and frusemide on blood pressure and plasma renin activity and electrolytes. *Br Heart J* 1985;53:611–615.
16. Gould BA, Hornung RS, Altman DG, Cashman PMM, Raftery EB. Indirect measurement of blood pressure during exercise testing can be misleading. *Postgrad Med J* 1976;52(suppl 7):119-122.
17. Gould BA, Hornung RS, Kieso HA, Cashman PMM, Raftery EB. An evaluation of self-recorded blood pressure during drug trials. *Hypertension* 1986; 8:267–271.
18. Gould BA, Kieso HA, Hornung RS, Altman DG, Cashman PMM, Raftery EB. Assessment of the accuracy and role of self-recorded blood pressures in the management of hypertension. *Br Med J* 1982;285:1691–1694.
19. Gould BA, Mann S, Davies AB, Altman DG, Raftery EB. Does placebo lower blood pressure. *Lancet* 1981;2:1377–1381.
20. Hahn LP, Folsom AR, Sprafka JM, Prineas RJ. Prevalence and accuracy of home sphygmomanometers in an urban population. *Am J Public Health* 1987; 77:1459–1461.
21. Jacot des Combes B, Porchet M, Waeber B, Brunner HR. Ambulatory blood pressure recordings: reproducibility and unpredictability. *Hypertension* 1984; 3:C110–C115.
22. James GD, Pickering TG, Yee LS, Harshfield GA, Riva S, Laragh JH. The reproducibility of average ambulatory, home, and clinic pressures. *Hypertension* 1988;11:545–549.
23. Kenny RA, Brennan M, O'Malley K, O'Brien E. Blood pressure measurements in borderline hypertension. *J Hypertens* 1987;5(suppl 5):483–485.
24. Kleinert HD, Harshfield GA, Pickering TG, Devereux RB, Sullivan PA, Marion RM, Mallory WK, Laragh JH. What is the value of home blood pressure measurement in patients with mild hypertension? *Hypertension* 1984;6:574–578.
25. Laughlin KD, Fisher L, Sherrard DJ. Blood pressure reductions during self-recording of home blood pressure. *Am Heart J* 1979;98:629–634.

26. Littler WA, Honour AJ, Pugsley DJ, Sleight P. The use of 24 hour blood pressure monitoring in the diagnosis and management of difficult hypertensive problems. *Postgrad Med J* 1976;52(suppl 52):119–122.
27. Littler WA, Honour AJ, Sleight P, Stott FD. Continuous recording of direct arterial pressure and electrocardiogram in unrestricted man. *Br Med J* 1972; 3:76–78.
28. Mancia G. Methods for assessing blood pressure values in humans. *Hypertension* 1983;5(suppl 3):5–13.
29. Mancia G, Bertinieri G, Grassi G, Pomidossi G, Gregorini L, Parati G, Ferrari A, Zanchetti A. Effects of blood pressure measurement by the doctor on patient's blood pressure and heart rate. *Lancet* 1983;2:695–698.
30. Marolf AP, Hany S, Bättig B, Vetter W. Comparison of casual, ambulatory and self-determined blood pressure measurement. *Nephron* 1987;47(suppl 1): 142–145.
31. McGrath BP, Beilin LJ, Schofield T, Benedict CR, Barker NP, Coomper R. Home blood pressure monitoring and changes in plasma catecholamines during once or twice daily treatment with atenolol in patients with mild hypertension. *Aust NZ J Med* 1979;9:374–381.
32. Mejia AD, Egan BM, Schork NJ, Zweifler AJ. Artefacts in measurement of blood pressure and lack of target organ involvement in the assessment of patients with treatment-resistant hypertension. *Ann Intern Med* 1990;112:270–277.
33. Ménard J, Serrurier D, Bautier P, Plouin PF, Corvol P. Crossover design to test antihypertensive drugs with self-recorded blood pressure. *Hypertension* 1988;11:153–159.
34. Memorandum from the WHO/ISH. 1986 Guidelines for the treatment of hypertension. *Hypertension* 1986;8:957–961.
35. O'Brien E, Mee F, Atkins N, O'Malley K. Inaccuracy of seven popular sphygmomanometers for home-measurement of blood pressure. *J Hypertens* 1990; 8:621–634.
36. O'Brien E, O'Malley K, Fitzgerald D. The role of home and ambulatory blood pressure recording in the management of hypertension. *J Hypertens* 1985; 3(suppl 1):35–39.
37. Padfield PL, Lindsay BA, McLaren JA, Pirie A, Rademarker M. Changing relation between home and clinic blood pressure measurements: Do home measurements predict clinic hypertension. *Lancet* 1987;2:322–324.
38. Parker D, Liu K, Dyer AR, Giumetti D, Liao Y, Stamler J. A comparison of the random-zero and standard mercury sphygmomanometers. *Hypertension* 1988;11:269–272.
39. Pickering TG. Blood pressure monitoring outside the office for the evaluation of patients with resistant hypertension. *Hypertension* 1988;11(Suppl 2):96–100.
40. Poggi L, Vaisse B, Bernard F, Agabriel P. Etude de l'effet placebo par mesure ambulatoire non sanglante de la pression artérielle. *Arch Mal Coeur* 1987; 80:1031–1036.
41. Porchet M, Bussien JP, Waeber B, Nussberger J, Brunner HR. Unpredictability of blood pressures recorded outside the clinic in the treated hypertensive patient. *J Cardiovasc Pharmacol* 1986;8:332–335.
42. Rion F, Waeber B, Graf HJ, Jaussi A, Porchet M, Brunner HR. Blood pres-

sure response to antihypertensive therapy: ambulatory versus office blood pressure readings. *J Hypertens* 1985;3:139–143,521.
43. Schaller MD, Nussberger J, Waeber B, Porchet M, Brunner HR. Transdermal clonidine therapy in hypertensive patients: effects on office and ambulatory recorded blood pressure values. *JAMA* 1985;253:233–235.
44. Streitberg B, Meyer-Sabellek W, Baumgart P. Statistical analysis of circadian blood pressure recordings in controlled clinical trials. *J Hypertens* 1989; 7(suppl 3):11–17.
45. Torriani S, Waeber B, Petrillo A, Di Stefano R, Mooser V, Scherrer U, Nussberger J, Hofstetter JR, Brunner HR. Usefulness of ambulatory blood pressure monitoring in the elderly hypertensive patient. *J Hypertens* 1988; 6(Suppl 1):25–27.
46. Van Egeren L. Repeated measurements of ambulatory blood pressure. *J Hypertens* 1988;6:753–755.
47. Waeber B, Avigdor L, Brunner HR. Long-term follow-up study of hypertensive patients by practicing internists after a controlled drug trial. *Clin Ther* 1984;6:509–515.
48. Waeber B, Burnier M, Perret F, Nussberger J, Brunner HR. Ambulatory blood pressure measurement and antihypertensive therapy. *J Hypertens* 1989;7(suppl 3):33–39.
49. Waeber B, Scherrer U, Petrillo A, Bidiville J, Nussberger J, Waeber G, Hofstetter JR, Brunner HR. Are some hypertensive patients overtreated? Results of a prospective study of ambulatory blood pressure recordings. *Lancet* 1987;2:732–734.
50. Waeber G, Beck G, Waeber B, Bidiville J, Nussberger J, Brunner HR. Comparison of betaxolol with verapamil in hypertensive patients: discrepancy between office and ambulatory blood pressures. *J Hypertens* 1988;6:239–245.
51. Watson RDS, Lumb R, Young MA, Stallard TJ, Davies P, Littler WA. Variation in cuff blood pressure in untreated outpatients with mild hypertension—Implications for initiating antihypertensive treatment. *J Hypertens* 1987; 5:207–211.
52. Weber MA. Whole-day blood pressure. AHA Focus Series. *Hypertension* 1989;3:35-45.
53. White WB. Methods of blood pressure determination to assess antihypertensive agents: Are casual measurements enough? *Clin Pharmacol Ther* 1989; 45:581–586.
54. White WB, McCabe EJ, Hager WD, Schulman P. The effects of the long-acting angiotensin-converting enzyme inhibitor cilazapril on casual, exercise and ambulatory blood pressure. *J Clin Pharmacol* 1988;44:173–178.
55. White WB, Morganroth J. Usefulness of ambulatory monitoring of blood pressure in assessing antihypertensive therapy. *Am J Cardiol* 1989;63:94–98.
56. World Hypertension League. Self-measurement of blood pressure: a statement by the World Hypertension League. *J Hypertens* 1988;6:257–261.

Ambulatory Blood Pressure Recording,
edited by H. Brunner and B. Waeber.
Raven Press, Ltd., New York © 1992.

8

A Pragmatic Look at Ambulatory Blood Pressure Monitoring

Hans R. Brunner, Bernard Waeber, and Jürg Nussberger

Hypertension Division and Cardiovascular Research Group, University Hospital, Lausanne, Switzerland

Ambulatory blood pressure measurement, based on invasive or, more importantly, noninvasive methods, has now been used for many years, has produced a host of interesting results and stirred a growing interest among physicians (1–4). Nevertheless, there is still no definitive agreement concerning its clinical usefulness and its precise indication for diagnostic purposes or for the evaluation of the efficacy of antihypertensive therapy (5,6).

It has to be kept in mind that the only justification for our interest in blood pressure measurement and hypertension is the knowledge that a rise in blood pressure enhances the risk of suffering a major cardiovascular complication such as stroke or heart attack (7). Accordingly, blood pressure measurement is not a goal in itself; blood pressure is only a substitute endpoint in an attempt to quantitate risk. Therefore, the usefulness of a new method to measure blood pressure can only be assessed by its accuracy in predicting risk. To better understand our approach to evaluating risk by measuring blood pressure, it may be interesting to compare it to the measurement of blood cholesterol, another indicator of cardiovascular risk.

Many prospective studies have shown that the shape of the curve relating cholesterol and blood pressure to the cardiovascular risk is almost identical (7,8). Measurements of blood pressure and total cholesterol in the serum are widely used in general practice to screen for patients with an enhanced risk of developing a myocardial infarction, a stroke, renal failure, or other cardiovascular complications. So far, several primary prevention trials have demonstrated the regression in coronary heart disease after the reduction of circulating total cholesterol (9–11), but lowering of blood pressure has been found to be less effective in decreasing the incidence of myocardial infarction (12,13). Before the initiation of costly and potentially hazardous treatment of a currently healthy person with the intention of preventing a hypothetical future disease, the physicians need persuasive arguments showing that active intervention will produce a clear benefit.

HOW GOOD ARE WE AT EVALUATING CARDIOVASCULAR RISK?

Blood pressure and total serum cholesterol levels are both biological variables that exhibit considerable variations. The measurement of blood pressure is still based on the indirect method using a sphygmomanometer and a stethoscope, and indeed most of the large trials so far have been carried out using this device, which has hardly changed during the last century. The measurement of blood pressure with this indirect method and the determination of total cholesterol have provided the basis for identifying these two variables as risk factors in large groups of patients (7,8). However, they have been less than satisfactory in predicting the risk in the individual patient. Particularly in younger subjects, blood pressure–related risk is very small, and it can therefore be questioned whether it is really sound reasoning that all subjects in whom a slight blood pressure elevation has been found need to be treated for the remainder of their life. This problem is still further confounded by the fact that blood pressure is highly variable and reproducibility of blood pressure measured casually by a physician is rather poor (14,15).

The cholesterol circulating in plasma does not flow in a free state but is packaged in lipoprotein particles. Thus, today it is possible to distinguish different lipoprotein fractions of cholesterol, and interest has concentrated on the high-density lipoprotein (HDL) and low-density lipoprotein (LDL) fractions (16). It was demonstrated that the risk for heart disease is inversely related to the HDL cholesterol

(17). The HDL cholesterol was subsequently recognized to play the role of a protective factor against the atherosclerotic process (18). Today the metabolic pathway of cholesterol is studied in even greater detail and this leads to a progressive refinement and an enhanced specificity in identifying patients with a truly increased risk.

In contrast, the blood pressure measuring techniques have not really evolved during recent years. In all major prospective trials, the measurement of blood pressure was made with a mercury sphygmomanometer using 1st and 5th Korotkoff sounds for the determination of systolic and diastolic blood pressure. However, it is well known that the blood pressure level is markedly, albeit to a variable degree, influenced by the presence of a physician (19). This phenomenon, usually called the "white-coat" effect or the alert reaction, can induce punctual blood pressure increases that often are around 10 to 15 mmHg but can go as high as 30 or even more mmHg (20–22). Is it reasonable to continue to use a method that yields such highly variable results? The answer seems to be clearly no, unless the goal of the blood pressure measurement is to evaluate the capacity of a patient to manage the stress represented by the measurement of blood pressure per se. This would be useful, if it were known that the blood pressure increase induced by the presence of the physician is an indicator of risk. There is today certainly little evidence available that this is so, and some of the evidence presented even makes this appear rather unlikely.

It is often argued that all the major trials that led to the recognition of blood pressure as a cardiovascular risk factor and all the major intervention trials providing evidence for risk reduction by antihypertensive therapy have been carried out using conventional blood pressure measurements obtained by a physician. Consequently, only the conventional blood pressure measuring method can be considered validated. In our opinion this reasoning is somewhat fallacious since these trials basically have only evaluated the relationship between blood pressure and risk and not a particular method of measuring blood pressure. Any measuring method, even if it is very inaccurate as our conventional method used, if it shows a weak correlation with the real variable, should also correlate with other factors related to the true variable, as long as a large enough number of subjects has been studied. Indeed all the risk evaluation and intervention trials have needed large numbers of patients to demonstrate small changes in risk, which in itself demonstrates the weakness of a conventionally measured blood pressure as an indicator of cardiovascular risk (12).

The important question then is, can we do better?

WHAT IS THE EVIDENCE THAT AMBULATORY BLOOD PRESSURE MONITORING PROVIDES ADVANTAGES?

The potential benefits that can be derived from ambulatory blood pressure monitoring are mainly due to two characteristics inherent to this method: (a) Many blood pressure measurements are available that can be treated with statistical methods to provide a blood pressure that more closely represents the true blood pressure prevailing during the day (23,24). (b) These blood pressure measurements are obtained when the patient pursues his usual activities, thus eliminating the stress involved in confronting his physician, that is, the stress caused by the obligation of facing his own health analysis.

The effect of these two characteristics is seen most directly when evaluating antihypertensive drugs in randomized trials. Many examples have illustrated this and the phenomenon has been analyzed to show beyond any doubt that with the appropriate design, the efficacy of drugs can be evaluated or compared using relatively small study populations with a much greater precision than using the conventional blood pressure measuring approach (25,26). If such an approach were used more widely for the development and evaluation of drugs, cost could be markedly reduced by reducing the size of the trials, and these savings would probably easily offset the additional cost introduced by the blood pressure recording (27). Furthermore, the scientific community would have the benefit of more clear-cut results in the literature.

As to the evaluation of cardiovascular risk, the evidence that ambulatory blood pressure recording may be more accurate in assessing this risk is still relatively limited (28). Nevertheless, the data that are available are all very encouraging. Thus, in a study that was at least partially prospective, it was found that patients with a high clinic pressure and a low ambulatory pressure had a better prognosis with regard to cardiovascular morbid events than those with a similar clinic pressure but a high ambulatory pressure (29,30). Several other studies have shown that ambulatory blood pressure correlated more closely than clinic pressure with left ventricular hypertrophy (31). Taken together, these studies strongly suggest that ambulatory blood pressure measurements may provide a higher degree of accuracy in predicting cardiovascular risk than casual blood pressure measured by the physician in his office.

The analysis of blood pressure profiles obtained during 24 hr could result in a few other benefits. It provides the possibility of analyzing, for instance, the antihypertensive effect of a given drug during a whole 24-hr period in order to determine if the dosing intervals of that drug have been chosen correctly (23). Nevertheless, such an analysis of trough versus peak antihypertensive effect of a drug can also be carried out by measuring the blood pressure manually just before dosing and at the time of the presumed peak effect. Such subanalysis of a blood pressure profile actually has the disadvantage of decreasing the statistical power of the blood pressure measurement by introducing a new dilution bias. More recently, it has also been suggested that analysis of the ambulatory blood pressure profile may provide a base to screen for secondary hypertension (32). In our opinion, it is still too early to recommend such an approach for general clinical use.

What is Deterring Us from Recommending Ambulatory Blood Pressure Monitoring for General Use?

First, there is the problem of normalcy. Indeed, so far there are very few cross-sectional data available on general and unselected populations (33,34). At the least, there is general agreement today that only in this way can normalcy be determined, and there is actually one such study in progress right now.

The question is if normalcy is such an important issue. The Framingham study has shown very clearly that the blood pressure distribution in the general population is a continuum stretching from what we consider "normal" to clearly hypertensive levels (7). Furthermore, the risk–blood pressure relationship is also continuous, such that risk decreases progressively down to the lowest blood pressure levels (7). In fact, normal values for the conventional method of measuring blood pressure have been quite arbitrarily limited to below 140/90 mmHg by the World Health Organization (WHO) (35).

There is really only one relevant question: Above which blood pressure level does the benefit of antihypertensive therapy exceed its untoward effects on cardiovascular risk? In spite of the WHO definition of a normal blood pressure for conventional blood pressure measuring techniques, this lower limit of blood pressure above which treatment should be initiated has been a matter of debate for many years and markedly different values have been proposed and are actually used in different countries. Thus, it has to be kept in mind that even using conventional blood pressure measurement, there is still considerable debate about who needs treatment in this largest subfraction of hypertensive patients, that is, those with only borderline blood pressure elevations (12,36,37).

This leads to the second problem: there are hardly any large trials available concerning blood pressure–risk relationships or risk reduction by antihypertensive therapy using ambulatory blood pressure recording. As a consequence, it is not absolutely clear today, based on ambulatory blood pressure recordings, which patient is at risk, who needs treatment, and how much risk reduction can be obtained by a given decrease in ambulatory blood pressure. Although this argument is correct, it is important to consider what can be done to obtain the necessary information. The Framingham study started more than 30 years ago (7). It is absolutely impossible today to start another study of the same type but based instead on ambulatory blood pressure recording. The world has changed, and it would be impossible to follow untreated patients for years in order to obtain risk profiles. For similar reasons, large therapeutic intervention trials based on ambulatory blood pressure recording with the goal of determining the limit, above which blood pressure needs to be treated, are very unlikely to become available for many years.

As scientists, we want to have facts before adopting new knowledge, concepts, or procedures. It has taken medicine a long time to adopt some scientific assessment principles, and we certainly do not want to advocate a departure from these. However, the present argument should be viewed from a different angle by concentrating on our generally accepted and widely used method of measuring blood pressure. Blood pressure measurement seems technically simple and straightforward. However, any pharmaceutical company knows the problems and difficulties of obtaining a clear dose-response curve for antihypertensive drugs. Our conventional blood pressure measuring technique, at least the way it is handled by most physicians, is not accurate enough to provide data needed to answer such a simple question. Reproducibility of blood pressure measurements is extremely poor (15). Furthermore, we know that blood pressure measured by the physician or a nurse can differ by a highly variable degree from the average blood pressures prevailing during the day (19–22). Even if we do not completely understand the physiological consequences of this alert reaction, we definitely know that in the physician's office very often a wrong impression is gained of the true blood pressure of the patient. Indeed, it would be very difficult to introduce such a method today with a new claim for accurate risk assessment to be used by every practicing physician. The fact is that risk assessment by conventional blood pressure measurement in the physician's office is evidently completely inadequate.

Why then do we still hold on to this inadequate method? We do so because the majority of the data on the blood pressure–risk relationship has been obtained with this approach. However, it should be remembered that this method has mostly proven its value in the early intervention trials studying patients with very high blood pressure and consequently high risk. It is not surprising that the more recent trials studying populations at much lower risk, and these represent the majority of our patients, have been disappointing in that, despite the large number of patients studied, only relatively small risk reductions could be demonstrated (12). Is it really appropriate to still hold on to a completely outdated method that we know is inaccurate, particularly the way it is handled in general practice, just because what promises to be a better method has not been proven in long prospective trials, which will probably never become available anyhow?

What are the Risks of Not Using Ambulatory Blood Pressure Monitoring?

Decisions of tremendous consequence for the remainder of the patient's life are taken based on a few blood pressure measurements, knowing very well that these may be quite erroneous. The patients are given the strong advice, and most of them are not able to resist it, to take every day one, two, or more drugs that may have beneficial effects, but that may in many cases be totally unnecessary and result only in untoward effects with no benefit. This is to say that based on the statistics available from the large intervention trials, probably only a small minority of our patients derive any benefit from therapy. That might be related to the lack of specificity of our methods used to identify cardiovascular risk. If we accept the concept that with a more specific method of identifying risk considerably fewer subjects would have to be exposed to pharmacological therapy, the present situation seems at least not very satisfactory. Unnecessary treatment not only causes iatrogenic morbidity, it also costs money. Of course, ambulatory blood pressure monitoring is still rather costly. With more general use, its price could certainly be reduced. More importantly, some of the cost would be offset by these savings from decreased drug use. However, whatever the cost of ambulatory blood pressure monitoring, no price is higher than that of a procedure that does not provide a clear benefit.

Similarly, if new antihypertensive agents continue to be developed using conventional blood pressure measurement, it will always remain difficult to obtain clear dose-response curves. As a consequence, drugs may continue to be used at excessive doses. Furthermore, because of the lack of accuracy of the method used, statistical power of the drug evaluation programs will be low and large numbers of subjects have to be studied. This again means higher developmental costs and higher prices burdening the health care programs.

CONCLUSION

The use of ambulatory blood pressure recordings has produced results that strongly suggest that this method may be superior to the conventional blood pressure measurement for the identification of cardiovascular risk and for evaluation of antihypertensive treatment. Because large prospective trials of ambulatory blood pressure monitoring are lacking, the use of this method has reached a plateau. However, it is unlikely that such data will become available in the near future. The important question is if the blood pressure measuring techniques used so far are good enough to warrant their continued use. We would like to argue that the results obtained with the conventional methods are much less convincing than generally claimed. Because of the inadequacy of the methods used so far, new approaches are badly needed. Ambulatory blood pressure recording has so far provided results that do suggest that it may be superior. We therefore believe that the time has come to give this method a serious try even though its definite superiority has not been proven but knowing that harder evidence can only be obtained with a more generalized use.

REFERENCES

1. Pickering TG, Harshfield GA, Devereux, RB, Laragh JH. What is the role of ambulatory blood pressure monitoring in the management of hypertensive patients? *Hypertension* 1985;7:171–177.
2. O'Brien E, Fitzgerald D, O'Malley K. Blood pressure measurement: current practice and future trends. *Br Med J* 1985;290:729–734.
3. Brunner HR, Waeber B, Nussberger J. Clinical use of non-invasive ambulatory blood pressure recording. *J Hypertens* 1985;3(Suppl 2):S13–S17.
4. White WB, Morganroth J. Usefulness of ambulatory monitoring of blood pressure in assessing antihypertensive therapy. *Am J Cardiol* 1989;63:94–98.
5. The Scientific Committee. Consensus document on non-invasive ambulatory blood pressure monitoring. *J Hypertens* 1990;8(Suppl 6):135–140.
6. The National High Blood Pressure Education Program Coordinating Committee. National high blood pressure education program working group report on ambulatory blood pressure monitoring. *Arch Intern Med* 1990;150:2270–2280.
7. Stokes J, Kannel WB, Wolf PA, D'Agostino RB, Cupples LA. Blood pressure as a risk factor for cardiovascular disease. The Framingham study—30 years of follow-up. *Hypertension* 1989;13(Suppl 1):I13–I18.
8. Martin MJ, Hulley SB, Browner WS, Kuller LH, Wentworth D. Serum cholesterol, blood pressure and mortality: Implications from a cohort of 361,662 men. *Lancet* 1986;2:933–936.
9. Lipid Research Clinics Program. The Lipid Research Clinics Coronary Primary Prevention Trial Results. I. Reduction in incidence of coronary heart disease. *JAMA* 1984;251:351–364.

10. Frick MH, Elo O, Haapa K, Heinonen OP, Heinsalmi P, Helo P, Huttunen JK, Kaitaniemi P, Koskinen P, Manninen V, Maenpaa H, Malkönen M, Mänttäri M, Norola S, Pasternack A, Pikkarainen J, Romo M, Sjöblom T, Nikkalä EA. Helsinki Heart Study: Primary prevention trial with gemfibrozil in middle-aged men with dyslipidemia. *N Engl J Med* 1987;317:1237–1245.
11. Canner PL, Berge KG, Wenger NK, Stamler L, Friedman RJP, Friedewold W. Fifteen year mortality in coronary drug project patients: long-term benefit with niacin. *J Am Coll Cardiol* 1986;8:1245–1255.
12. Cutler JA, MacMahon SW, Furberg CD. Controlled clinical trials of drug treatment for hypertension. A review. *Hypertension* 1989;13(Suppl 1):I36–I44.
13. Cruickshank JM, Thorp JM, Zacharias FJ. Benefits and potential harm of lowering high blood pressure. *Lancet* 1987;1;581–584.
14. Richardson DW, Honour AJ, Fenton GW, Stott FH, Pickering GW. Variation in arterial pressure throughout the day and night. *Clin Sci* 1964;26:445–460.
15. Coats AJS. Reproducibility or variability of casual and ambulatory blood pressure data: implications for clinical trials. *J Hypertens* 1990;8(Suppl 6):17–20.
16. Hulley SB, Roads GG. The plasma lipoproteins as risk factors: Comparison of electrophoretic and ultracentrifugation results. *Metabolism* 1982;31:773–778.
17. Miller GJ, Miller NE. Plasma-high-density-lipoprotein concentration and development of ischaemic heart disease. *Lancet* 1975;1:16–19.
18. Gordon T, Castelli WP, Hjortland MC, Kannel WB, Dawber TR. High density lipoprotein as a protective factor against coronary heart disease. *Am J Med* 1977;62:707–714.
19. Mancia G, Bertinieri G, Grassi G, Pomidossi G, Gregorini L, Parati G, Ferrari A, Zanchetti A. Effects of blood pressure measurement by the doctor on patient's blood pressure and heart rate. *Lancet* 1983;2:695–698.
20. Floras JS, Jones JV, Hassan MO, Osikowska B, Sever PS, Sleight P. Cuff and ambulatory pressure in subjects with essential hypertension. *Lancet* 1981; 2:107–109.
21. Jacot des Combes B, Porchet M, Waeber B, Brunner HR. Ambulatory blood pressure recordings: reproducibility and unpredictability. *Hypertension* 1984; 3:C110–C115.
22. Porchet M, Bussien JP, Waeber B, Nussberger J, Brunner HR. Unpredictability of blood pressures recorded outside the clinic in the treated hypertensive patient. *J Cardiovasc Pharmacol* 1986;8:332–335.
23. White WB, Analysis of ambulatory blood pressure data in antihypertensive drug trials. *J Hypertens* 19991;9(Suppl 1):27–32.
24. Parati G, Mutti E, Ravogli A, Trazzi S, Villani A, Mancia G. Advantages and disadvantages of non-invasive ambulatory blood pressure monitoring. *J Hypertens* 1990;8(Suppl 6):33–38.
25. Waeber B, Nussberger J, Brunner HR. Are surgery blood pressure measurements adequate to evaluate the efficacy of antihypertensive drugs. *J Hypertens* 1984;2:449–451.
26. Conway J, Johnston J, Coats A, Somers V, Sleight P. The use of ambulatory blood pressure monitoring to improve the accuracy and reduce the numbers of subjects in clinical trials of antihypertensive agents. *J Hypertens* 1988;6:111–116.
27. Sheps SG. Cost considerations of ambulatory blood pressure monitoring. *J Hypertens* 1990;8(Suppl 6):29–31.

28. Brunner HR, Waeber B, Nussberger J. Blood pressure recording in the ambulatory patient and evaluation of cardiovascular risk. *Clin Sci* 1985;68:485–488.
29. Perloff D, Sokolow M, Cowan R. The prognostic value of ambulatory blood pressure. *JAMA* 1983;249:2792–2798.
30. Perloff D, Cowan RM, Juster RP. Prognostic value of ambulatory blood pressure measurements: further analysis. *J Hypertens* 1989;7(suppl 3):3–10.
31. Devereux RB, Pickering TG. Relationship between ambulatory or exercise blood pressure and left ventricular structure: prognostic implications. *J Hypertens* 1990;8(Suppl 6):125–134.
32. Imai Y, Abe K, Munakata M, Sakuma H, Hashimoto J, Imai K, Sekino H, Yoshinaga K. Does ambulatory blood pressure monitoring improve the diagnosis of secondary hypertension? *J Hypertens* 1990;8(Suppl 6):71–75.
33. Staessen J, Fagard R, Lijnen P, Thijs L, Van Hoof R, Amery A. Reference values for ambulatory blood pressure: a meta-analysis. *J Hypertens* 1990; 8(Suppl 6):57–64.
34. Cox J, O'Malley K, Atkins N, O'Brien E. A comparison of the twenty-four-hour blood pressure profile in normotensive and hypertensive subjects. *J Hypertens* 1991;9(Suppl 1):3–6.
35. Organisation Mondiale de la Santé. Hypertension artérielle et cardiopathies ischémiques. Serie de Rapports techniques 231, 1962.
36. Sleight P. When and how far should we lower blood pressure? *Hypertension* 1983;5(suppl 3):14–16.
37. Alderman MH, Madhavan S. Management of the hypertensive patient: a continuing dilemma. *Hypertension* 1981;3:192–197.

Subject Index

C

D

I

J